# WHAT YOU MUST KNOW ABOUT
# WOMEN'S HORMONES

## YOUR GUIDE TO NATURAL HORMONE TREATMENT FOR PMS, MENOPAUSE, OSTEOPOROSIS, PCOS, AND MORE

## PAMELA WARTIAN SMITH, MD, MPH

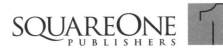

SQUAREONE
PUBLISHERS

EDITOR: Michele D'Altorio
COVER DESIGNER: Jeannie Tudor
TYPESETTER: Gary A. Rosenberg and Terry Wiscovitch

The information and advice contained in this book are based upon the research and the personal and professional experiences of the author. They are not intended as a substitute for consulting with a healthcare professional. The publisher and author are not responsible for any adverse effects or consequences resulting from the use of any of the suggestions, preparations, or procedures discussed in this book. All matters pertaining to your physical health should be supervised by a healthcare professional. It is a sign of wisdom, not cowardice, to seek a second or third opinion.

**Square One Publishers**
115 Herricks Road
Garden City Park, NY 11040
(516) 535-2010 • (877) 900-BOOK
www.squareonepublishers.com

**Library of Congress Cataloging-in-Publication Data**

Smith, Pamela Wartian.
  What you must know about women's hormones : your guide to natural hormone treatment for PMS, menopause, osteoporosis, PCOS, and more / Pamela Wartian Smith.
      p. cm.
  Includes bibliographical references and index.
  ISBN 978-0-7570-0307-3
  1. Menopause—Hormone therapy—Popular works. 2. Middle-aged women—Diseases—Hormone therapy—Popular works. 3. Endocrine gynecology--Popular works.  I. Title.
  RG186.S678 2009
  618.1'7506--dc22

                                2009040771

Printed in Canada

10   9   8   7   6   5   4   3   2   1

# Contents

## Part III:  Hormone Replacement Therapy

*To my daughters, Autumn, Hollie, and Caitlin,*
*and my step-daughters, Lynn and Sarah,*
*who are now just learning the importance*
*of optimal hormonal function.*

*To my husband Christopher,*
*whose patience with me as I traveled along*
*my own hormonal "journey"*
*has been nothing short of wonderful.*

# Acknowledgments

To my publisher, Rudy Shur, without whom this book would not be possible. His belief in my message was instrumental in making this book the best it can be.

I would also like to thank my editor, Michele D'Altorio, for her hard work and dedication to this project.

To Dr. Shari Lieberman, who has been instrumental in teaching me the primary role nutrition plays in overall health. Over the years, I have had the privilege of being able to call Dr. Lieberman my friend. My mother was right. You are very lucky in your life if you have five true friends. Dr. Lieberman is such a friend, as well as an internationally-known speaker, educator, and author. Her footprint on the future of Anti-Aging medicine will always remain.

# Preface

With the completion of the Genome Project, medicine has changed. The science is now here to individualize treatment—this includes hormonal therapies. How you metabolize medication, including hormones, or the amount you need are very different from your mother, your sister, or your friend.

Much of this book is written in a concise, bullet-style format, as opposed to long, literary prose. It was formatted as such for today's busy woman who does not want to wade through extraneous sentence structure. You can see the important points at a moment's glance. Consequently, many of the lengthy scientific explanations are not present in the body of this text. For those readers who want a further explanation of the principles contained in this book, please avail yourself of the numerous citations from the medical journals in the References section.

There is also a Summaries section at the back of the book that lists important points from each chapter in a short, concise, easy-to-locate manner, also designed for reader convenience.

It is my hope that this book will serve as a reference for all women so that we can each receive the individualized care that we all deserve.

In good health,

Pamela W. Smith, MD, MPH

# Introduction

**H**ow would you like to live to be 100 years old? Well, perhaps you can. We now have the scientific means to help you live to be at least 100 years of age, if not older. However, in order to live to that age, you need to be hormonally and nutritionally sound. I hope that my book will help you to achieve this. It was written to provide you with the hormonal aspects of staying healthy, along with a few nutritional aspects.

All the hormones in the body are a symphony. Much like an orchestra must play in tune, your hormonal symphony must be in tune throughout your life in order for you to have optimal health. Hormonal dysfunction can occur at any age—it is not exclusive to older people. For example, if you have PMS, postpartum depression, fibroids, or fibrocystic breast disease, there is a good chance that your progesterone-to-estrogen ratio is too low.

Treatment for these kinds of ailments (or any hormonal abnormality, for that matter) may involve hormone replacement therapy (HRT). In the past, no matter what her symptoms or hormonal levels were, every woman would receive the same one-size-fits-all treatment. Today, things are different.

This brings me to my second reason for writing this book: to herald a new age in medicine. With the completion of the Genome Project, a thirteen-year study completed in 2003 that was designed to identify the over 20,000 genes in human DNA, we now have the medical capability to develop and customize a treatment plan for each patient.

Medicine is at a crossroads. Now, instead of just treating the symptoms of a disease, a new model of medicine is emerging that looks at the cause of the problem. For example: why might a person suffer from depression? Antidepressants are wonderful medications—if you need them. Their purpose is to treat the symptoms of depression—not to uncover the cause of depression. In the new specialty of Metabolic/Anti-Aging Medicine, the reason *why* a person has depression would be looked at. Depression may be a symptom of hypothyroidism, which is low thyroid function. Or, it may be a result of the sufferer's body no longer making

1

enough estrogen, progesterone, or testosterone. There are many different factors that can cause depression, and Metabolic/Anti-Aging Medicine aims to find and alleviate the cause instead of just treating the various symptoms. Just because two people are suffering the same symptoms does not mean they should receive the same treatment. Metabolic/Anti-Aging Medicine recognizes this and treats patients accordingly. To find a Metabolic/Anti-Aging specialist, see the Resources section.

The pages of this text will explore the intricate web of your body's hormonal system, tying together my reasons for writing the book by explaining the hormonal aspects of staying healthy and examining how individualized HRT can prevent some ailments from occurring.

Part I of the text looks at the different hormones in your body, their functions, and the different side effects that can occur if these hormones are not at optimal levels. Additionally, the importance of hormonal levels and the ratio between them will be revealed. You will also learn the different etiologies that can cause hormonal imbalances, which may help you eliminate a problem before it gets too serious. The correct levels of all of your hormones are needed for you to achieve optimal health.

I have organized Part I, the hormones, in the order I felt would be most useful to women. While the order of importance for every woman may be different, understanding each hormone is key.

Part II focuses on the most common ailments and problems that arise from hormonal imbalances, such as perimenopause and menopause, PMS, postpartum depression, and endometriosis, to name a few. You'll learn that even diseases that seemingly have nothing to do with hormones—like heart disease and osteoporosis—can be affected by a hormonal imbalance. Keeping your hormones at optimal levels is beneficial in preventing an array of ailments, even ones you wouldn't suspect.

Part III focuses on HRT. You'll learn the difference between synthetic and natural HRT, and how to get started should you decide HRT is the option for you. Different ways to have your hormone levels measured are discussed, along with a few examples of HRT. Finally, you will learn how proper nutrition can benefit and boost the effects of HRT.

Fortunately, we do not have to suffer in silence like our mothers did! Science can help us. Not only can we have our symptoms resolved, but we now have a better chance of helping maintain our vision, memory, and mobility. This is not "Star Trek" medicine. It is here and available now. You too can have individualized and customized care. This book will help you discover how.

# PART I

---

# Hormones

# Introduction to Part I

The hormones in your body are a key component of your overall health. A hormone is a chemical substance produced in the body that controls and regulates the activity of certain cells or organs. All the hormones in your body interact with each other. They are a web; a symphony that must play in tune in order for you to feel great and be healthy.

This part of the book looks at many of the hormones in your body. Your sex hormones—estrogen, progesterone, testosterone, and DHEA— will be explored. The importance of having a balanced ratio between these hormones will also be discussed.

Your sex hormones interact with cortisol (your stress hormone) and insulin (your glucose regulator). All of these hormones (besides insulin) are made by pregnenolone, your memory hormone. Our sex hormones are what make us women. They literally play as a symphony in the body. If your hormonal symphony is playing in tune, you feel fabulous. If your hormones are not balanced (playing out of tune), you will experience symptoms.

Additionally, these hormones all interact with your thyroid hormone, which regulates many important functions in your body, including metabolism. Just like the ratio between your sex hormones is important, thyroid levels that are too high or too low can have serious consequences, which will also be discussed in this section of the book.

Your hormone levels change throughout your lifetime. The amount of hormones your body makes and the degree of fluctuation or change in hormone levels is important. There are many things that influence how much of a hormone is made. For example, if you are stressed, take an antibiotic, deliver a baby, are near toxins, have an unhealthy diet, exercise too much or not enough, or take too few or too many vitamins, the amount of hormones that your body produces will be affected.

As mentioned in the Introduction to the book, I chose to organize the sections in Part I by order of importance instead of alphabetical order. This is the order of importance in a woman's body when symptoms, diseases, and other hormonal issues are taken into consideration. Of course, different women have different hormonal needs, and this order will not be the order of importance for every single woman. But, it is the *overall* order of importance.

Let us begin our hormonal journey.

# ESTROGEN

Estrogen is a female hormone that is produced in the ovaries. Your body has receptor cites for estrogen everywhere: in your brain, muscles, bone, bladder, gut, uterus, ovaries, vagina, breasts, eyes, heart, lungs, and blood vessels, to name a few. Estrogen has over 400 crucial functions in your body. It regulates your body temperature, helps prevent Alzheimer's disease, helps prevent muscle damage and maintain muscles, helps regulate your blood pressure, enhances your energy, improves your mood, and increases your sexual interest.

## ■ Other Functions of Estrogen in Your Body

- Acts as a natural calcium blocker to keep your arteries open
- Aids in the formation of neurotransmitters in your brain—such as serotonin—which decrease depression, irritability, anxiety, and pain sensitivity
- Decreases LDL (bad cholesterol) and prevents its oxidation
- Decreases lipoprotein A (a risk factor for heart disease)
- Decreases the accumulation of plaque on your arteries
- Decreases wrinkles
- Decreases your risk of developing colon cancer
- Dilates your small arteries
- Enhances magnesium uptake and utilization
- Enhances the production of nerve-growth factor
- Helps maintain the elasticity of your arteries
- Helps maintain your memory

- Helps prevent tooth loss
- Helps with fine motor skills
- Improves insulin sensitivity
- Increases blood flow
- Increases concentration
- Increases HDL (good cholesterol) by 10 to 15 percent
- Increases reasoning
- Increases the water content of your skin, which is responsible for your skin's thickness and softness
- Increases your metabolic rate, which helps your body run at a youthful level
- Inhibits platelet stickiness, which decreases your risk of heart disease
- Maintains bone density
- Maintains the amount of collagen in your skin
- Protects you against macular degeneration, an age-related eye ailment that may cause vision loss

- Reduces homocysteine (a risk factor for heart disease)
- Reduces your overall risk of heart disease by 40 to 50 percent
- Reduces vascular proliferation and inflammatory responses, which decrease your risk of heart disease
- Reduces your risk of cataracts

Estrogen levels are lower in women who smoke. This may be why women who smoke have more menopausal symptoms than women who do not smoke. Also, low-fat diets decrease free estrogen (the amount of estrogen available for your body to use).

### ■ Symptoms of Estrogen Deficiency

- ☐ Acne
- ☐ Anxiety
- ☐ Arthritis
- ☐ Bladder problems (more infections, urinary leakage)
- ☐ Brittle hair and nails
- ☐ Chronic fatigue syndrome
- ☐ Decrease in breast size
- ☐ Decrease in dexterity
- ☐ Decrease in memory
- ☐ Decrease in sexual interest/function
- ☐ Depression
- ☐ Diabetes
- ☐ Difficulty losing weight, even with diet and exercise
- ☐ Dry eyes
- ☐ Elevated blood pressure
- ☐ Elevated cholesterol
- ☐ Food cravings
- ☐ Fibromyalgia
- ☐ Heart attacks
- ☐ Increase in facial hair
- ☐ Increase in insulin resistance, which can lead to diabetes
- ☐ Increase in tension headaches
- ☐ Increased cholesterol
- ☐ Infertility
- ☐ Joint pain
- ☐ Low energy, especially at the end of the day
- ☐ More frequent migraines
- ☐ More wrinkles (aging skin)
- ☐ Oily skin
- ☐ Osteoporosis/osteopenia
- ☐ Panic attacks
- ☐ Polycystic ovarian syndrome
- ☐ Restless sleep
- ☐ Stress incontinence
- ☐ Strokes
- ☐ Thinner skin
- ☐ Thinning hair
- ☐ Urinary tract infections
- ☐ Vaginal dryness
- ☐ Vulvodynia (vaginal pain)
- ☐ Weight gain around the middle

Most women who suffer estrogen-related problems are estrogen dominant. However, even though it is less common, women can also have estrogen deficiencies. There are only two causes of estrogen deficiency.

## ■ Causes of Estrogen Deficiency

- Perimenopause and menopause
- Premature ovarian decline

As mentioned, most women with estrogen issues have too much estrogen in their bodies. Dr. John Lee coined the phrase "estrogen dominance" to describe the symptoms of excess estrogen in the body.

Estrogen dominance can result from the overproduction of estrogen or from the progesterone-estrogen ratio not being balanced. If you're experiencing symptoms of estrogen excess, it may also be the result of how the body breaks down estrogen.

## ■ Symptoms of Excess Estrogen

- ☐ Bloating
- ☐ Cervical dysplasia
- ☐ Decrease in sexual interest
- ☐ Depression with anxiety or agitation
- ☐ Elevated risk of developing breast cancer
- ☐ Fatigue
- ☐ Fibrocystic breasts
- ☐ Headaches
- ☐ Heavy periods
- ☐ Hypothyroidism (increases the binding of thyroid hormone, which causes low thyroid hormone levels)
- ☐ Increased risk of developing autoimmune diseases
- ☐ Increased risk of developing uterine cancer
- ☐ Irritability
- ☐ Mood swings
- ☐ Panic attacks
- ☐ Poor sleep
- ☐ Swollen breasts
- ☐ Uterine fibroids (non-cancerous tumors of the uterus)
- ☐ Water retention
- ☐ Weight gain (especially in the abdomen, hips, and thighs)

## ■ Causes of Excess Estrogen

- Diet low in grains and fiber
- Elevation of 16-hydroxyestrone

- Environmental estrogens
- Impaired elimination of estrogen
- Lack of exercise
- Taking too much estrogen

## NATURAL ESTROGENS

"Natural" means biologically identical to the chemical structure that your own body makes. Your body makes many kinds of estrogen. The three main estrogens are E1, called estrone; E2, called estradiol; and E3, called estriol.

### Estrone (E1)

Estrone is the main estrogen your body produces post-menopausally. It is derived from estradiol (E2). High levels of E1 stimulate breast and uterine tissue, and many researchers believe this increases your risks for developing breast and uterine cancer.

E1 is considered a reserve source for estrogen. This is its only known function. If your estrogen levels get too low, your body can draw from and use this stored amount.

Before menopause, E1 is made by your ovaries, adrenal glands, liver, and fat cells. It is converted to E2 in your ovaries. Post-menopausally, very little E1 becomes E2, since the ovaries stop working. In later years, E1 is made in your fat cells and, to a lesser degree, in your liver and adrenal glands. Therefore, the more body fat you have, the more E1 you make. Consequently, obese women have an increased E1-to-E2 ratio. Also, routine alcohol consumption decreases ovarian hormone levels and increases your levels of E1, which can lead to an increased risk of breast cancer.

### Estradiol (E2)

Estradiol is the strongest form of estrogen. It is twelve times stronger than E1, and eighty times stronger than estriol (E3). It is the main estrogen your body produces before menopause. Most of your body's E2 is made in your ovaries. High levels of E2 are associated with an increased risk of breast and uterine cancer.

### ▣ Functions of E2 in Your Body

- Decreases fatigue
- Decreases LDL (bad cholesterol)
- Decreases platelet stickiness
- Decreases total cholesterol

- Decreases triglycerides (transdermal, on the skin, administration of E2 only)
- Helps maintain memory
- Helps maintain potassium levels
- Helps maintain your bones
- Helps with the absorption of calcium, magnesium, and zinc
- Improves sleep
- Increases endorphins
- Increases growth hormone
- Increases HDL (good cholesterol)
- Increases serotonin
- Works as an antioxidant

E2 is the form of estrogen you lose at menopause. However, two-thirds of postmenopausal women up to the age of eighty continue to make some E2. Women who have had a surgical procedure that affected their ovaries tend to have lower levels of E2 than other women. (See the section on surgical menopause, page 102.)

## ■ Symptoms of E2 Decline in Menstruating Women

- ☐ Aching joints
- ☐ Anxiety attacks that get worse around menstrual cycle
- ☐ Bladder changes, such as more infections, pain during urination, more frequent urination, and urinary leakage
- ☐ Bone loss in spine, resulting in slumped posture
- ☐ Decline in collagen, resulting in dry, crawly, looser skin and more wrinkles
- ☐ Difficulty having an orgasm
- ☐ Difficulty losing weight, even with diet and exercise
- ☐ Dry, brittle nails
- ☐ Dry eyes
- ☐ Fibromyalgia pain syndrome
- ☐ Food cravings
- ☐ Increase in facial hair
- ☐ Increase in tension headaches
- ☐ Loss of energy, or feeling too tired to get through the day
- ☐ Loss of sexual interest
- ☐ Memory and concentration problems that are worse before menstruation
- ☐ Mood swings, episodic tearfulness for no reason, irritability, angry outbursts, and spells of depression, especially premenstrually
- ☐ More irritable bowel problems prior to and during menstruation
- ☐ Muscle soreness or stiffness
- ☐ Palpitations, especially those that get worse a few days prior to menstruation and during the cycle
- ☐ Premenstrual migraines, or more frequent migraines

☐ Restless sleep, difficulty sleeping (especially prior to menstruating), or multiple awakenings during the night

☐ Spiking blood pressure, or blood pressure that is higher than your normal

☐ Thinner hair and more scalp hair loss

☐ Vaginal dryness, resulting in pain during intercourse

☐ Weight gain around the middle

☐ Worsening allergies, such as sensitivities to chemicals or perfumes

☐ Worsening PMS

## Estriol (E3)

Estriol (E3) has a much lesser stimulatory effect on the breast and uterine lining than E1 or E2. E3 does not promote breast cancer. In fact, considerable evidence exists to show that it protects against breast cancer. In Western Europe, E3 has been used for this purpose for over sixty years.

Estrogen has two main receptor sites that it binds to in the body: estrogen receptor-alpha and estrogen receptor-beta. Estrogen receptor-alpha increases cell growth and estrogen receptor-beta decreases cell growth and helps prevent breast cancer development. E2 equally activates estrogen receptors alpha and beta. E1 activates estrogen receptor-alpha selectively in a ratio of five-to-one. Therefore, E1 prefers to bind with the alpha receptor type, which increases cell proliferation. In contrast, E3 binds preferentially to estrogen receptor-beta in a three-to-one ratio. It is believed that this selective binding to estrogen-beta receptor sites imparts to E3 a potential for breast cancer prevention.

One of the wonderful things about E3 is that is an adaptogen, meaning it adapts to the specific environment of the body it is in. When given by itself, E3 does exert strong estrogenic effects. When given in a tenfold amount in relationship to E2, E3 antagonizes the effect of E2, and may also be another reason E3 helps decrease the risk of breast cancer.

Studies over the last thirty years have revealed that E3 given experimentally to women with breast cancer has decreased a reoccurrence of the disease. This includes one study in the 1970s where women with metastatic breasts were given E3. Of the women, 37 percent experienced remission—their cancer did not spread any further.

However, E3 does not have the bone, heart, or brain protection that E2 does. E3 does, however, have some positive effects on bone and also heart health by lowering cholesterol.

I usually begin by prescribing 20 percent E2 and 80 percent E3 for an estrogen prescription if tests reveal that a patient's estrogen levels are low. Then, the percentages of E2 and E3 are adjusted according to lab results of each patient. The combination of E2 and E3 together is called "biest," which is a prescription that a compounding pharmacist (a pharmacist who puts together medications in customized dosages) can formulate for you. Any percentage of these two estrogens can be used, since the dosage is personalized.

### ■ Functions of E3 in Your Body

- Benefits the vaginal lining
- Blocks E1 by occupying the estrogen receptor sites on your breast cells
- Controls symptoms of menopause, including hot flashes, insomnia, and vaginal dryness
- Decreases LDL (bad cholesterol)
- Helps reduce pathogenic bacteria
- Helps restore the proper pH of the vagina, which prevents urinary tract infections (UTIs)
- Helps your gut maintain a favorable environment for the growth of good bacteria (lactobacilli)
- Increases HDL (good cholesterol)

Before you begin HRT, it is necessary that you have your levels of all three estrogens measured. You should also have them measured regularly thereafter, to help your doctor ensure you maintain the optimal amount of each type of estrogen.

## SYNTHETIC ESTROGEN

Estrogen replacement comes in many forms. The most commonly prescribed hormone replacement in the United States is Premarin, which is a mixture of estrone (E1), sodium equilin sulfate, and concomitant components, such as 17 alpha-dihydroequilin, 17 alpha-estradiol, and 17 beta-dihydroequilin. It comes in pill form, and is commonly referred to as "synthetic estrogen."

Premarin contains horse estrogens (equilin and equilenin) and additives that are synthetic. These additives and coatings may cause their own side effects, including burning in the urinary tract, allergies, joint aches, and pains.

Synthetic estrogens contain many forms of estrogen that do not fit into the estrogen receptors in your body. It is unknown what happens to the estrogens that do not fit into your receptors.

The estradiol (E2) molecules your body makes are eliminated from your body through urine within a day. Conversely, equilin (estrogen

# Estrogen Detoxification

Estrogen synthesis, estrogen metabolism, and estrogen detoxification are of paramount importance in order to maintain optimal health. The effect of estrogen on your body is not related solely to its function but also to how it is detoxified in the liver and in other tissues.

Toxins are poisonous substances that are either produced by the body, inhaled, or ingested. When they build up, the heath effects can be quite serious. This is why it is important to detoxify.

Detoxification is the process through which toxic substances—environmental pollutants, medications, byproducts of metabolism, and more—are removed from the body. This process is one of the major functions of the liver, gastrointestinal tract, kidneys, and skin, with the liver being one of the most important organs of detoxification. Studies have shown that each individual has a different ability to break down toxins.

Each year, over 2.5 billion pounds of pesticides are dumped on crop lands, forests, lawns, and fields. According to the U.S. Environmental Protection Agency, more than 4 billion pounds of chemicals were released into the ground in the year 2000, threatening our natural ground water sources.

## Toxin Buildup

### ■ Symptoms of Toxin Buildup

| ☐ Fatigue | ☐ Headaches | ☐ Muscle aches and pains |
|---|---|---|

Toxicity also can affect your endocrine, immune, and neurological systems.

- Endocrine toxicity affects reproduction, menstruation, libido, metabolic rate, stress tolerance, and glucose regulation.

- Immune toxicity may be a factor in asthma, allergies, skin disorders, chronic infections, and cancer.

- Neurological toxicity also affects cognition, mood, and neurological function.

Finally, there are some activities and habits that increase your exposure to toxins. See the list below for some examples.

## ■ Your Exposure to Toxins is Increased by:

- Chronic use of medication(s)
- Drinking tap water
- Excessive consumption of alcohol
- Excessive consumption of caffeine
- Excessive consumption of processed foods and fats
- Intestinal (gut) dysfunction
- Kidney problems
- Lack of exercise

- Liver dysfunction
- Living or working near areas of high traffic of industrial plants
- Occupational or other exposure to pesticides, paints, and other toxic substances without adequate protective equipment
- Recreational drug use
- Tobacco use
- Using pesticides, paint, and other toxic substances without adequate protective gear

Every day, you are exposed to estrogen-like compounds. These are called "xenoestrogens." Xenoestrogens are environmental compounds with estrogenic activity, and can interfere with or mimic your own hormone synthesis. Consequently, they are disruptive to your own hormone production.

## The Detoxification Process

Detoxification is a process by which your body transforms toxins and medications into harmless molecules that can be eliminated. This process takes place primarily in the liver and to a smaller degree in other tissues, such as your gastrointestinal tract, skin, kidneys, and lungs.

Detoxification by the liver is largely accomplished in two phases. In Phase I, enzymes change toxins into intermediate compounds. In Phase II, the intermediate compounds are neutralized through the addition of a water-soluble molecule. The body is then able to eliminate the transformed toxins through the urine or feces.

It is very important for you to detoxify estrogen completely in your body. This is accomplished through Phase I and Phase II detoxification.

The next two pages will provide a more detailed description of Phase I and Phase II detoxification.

## PHASE I DETOXIFICATION:
## YOUR FIRST LINE OF DEFENSE

In Phase I detoxification, enzymes in the cytochrome P450 system use oxygen to modify toxic compounds, medications, and steroid hormones. This is your first line of defense for the detoxification of all environmental toxins, medications, supplements (for example, vitamins), and many waste products that your body produces.

The cytochrome P450 system is a group of over sixty enzymes that your body uses to break down toxins. Most of these enzymes are located in your liver. Three of the twelve cytochrome P450 gene families share the main responsibility for drug metabolism in your body. In other words, many of the medications that you take are broken down through this system. The cytochrome P450 system is also involved in other processes in your body, such as the conversion of vitamin D into more active forms.

Phase I occurs in the liver, where estrogen goes through the cytochrome P450 system. This influences the amount of estrogen that is exposed to your other cells. If you do not completely detoxify the intermediates of estrogen metabolism, it can result in an increase in estrogen activity in your body.

Within your own genetic makeup, there are variations called "single nucleotide polymorphisms" (SNPs, pronounced "snips"). These SNPs in your genes code for a particular enzyme that can increase or decrease the activity of that enzyme. Both increased and decreased activity may be harmful to you. Furthermore, if you have increased Phase I clearance (alimination) without increased Phase II clearance, this can lead to the buildup of intermediates that may be more toxic than the original substance.

Decreased Phase I clearance will cause toxic accumulation in your body. Sometimes, the body completes Phase I but builds up a toxic metabolite that Phase II is unable to eliminate from the system. Adverse reactions to medications are often due to a decreased capacity for clearing them from your system.

### ■ Nutrients Required for Phase I Detoxification

| | | |
|---|---|---|
| • Copper | • Niacin | • Vitamin $B_{12}$ |
| • Flavonoids | • Vitamin $B_2$ | • Vitamin C |
| • Folic acid | • Vitamin $B_3$ | • Zinc |
| • Magnesium | • Vitamin $B_6$ | |

## PHASE II DETOXIFICATION: CONJUGATION OF TOXINS AND ELIMINATION

In Phase II detoxification, large water-soluble molecules are added to toxins, usually at the reactive site formed by Phase I reactions. After Phase II modifications, the body is able to eliminate the transformed toxins in the urine or the feces. Phase II detoxification has six stages.

*Stage I:* Glutathione conjugation. Glutathione is the strongest antioxidant that your body makes. This stage of detoxification requires glutathione and vitamin $B_6$.

*Stage II:* Amino acid conjugation. This stage requires glycine, taurine, and glutamine.

*Stage III:* Methylation. Methylation is needed for many reactions in the body including detoxification of estrogen and breakdown of homocysteine. It requires folic acid, choline, methionine, trimethylglycine, and s-adenosylmethionine (SAMe).

*Stage IV:* Sulfation. Requires cysteine, methionine, and molybdenum.

*Stage V:* Acetylation. Requires acetyl CoA.

*Stage VI:* Glucuronidation. Requires glucuronic acid.

Phase I and Phase II detoxification can be measured. The test that does this analyzes saliva, blood, and urine after taking a challenge dose of caffeine, aspirin, and acetaminophen. The results reveal if there are any missing enzymes that are used to process these substances. If there are missing enzymes, they can be identified and replenished.

derived from the urine of horses) has been shown to stay in the body for up to thirteen weeks. This is due to the fact that your enzymes are designed to metabolize your own estrogen, and not equilin.

How you take estrogen is also important. I recommend only taking estrogen by the transdermal route, which means applying it to the skin.

### ■ Side Effects of Taking Estrogen Orally (Instead of Transdermally)

- Decrease in growth hormone (the hormone that keeps you younger)
- Elevated liver enzymes

# Genovations Testing

It is also possible to evaluate genetic variations that affect Phase I and Phase II detoxification and oxidative protection (the ability to get rid of free radical production). This genetically-based test is called "Genovations" and it is available through Genova Diagnostic Laboratory (see Resources on page 183 for more information). Through this kind of testing, your healthcare practitioner can determine early-on if the detoxification system in your body is working by identifying potential genetic trouble spots in your self-defense system. Then, if problem areas are detected, your doctor can design precise, individualized therapy to support your detoxification.

## ■ Benefits of Genovations Testing

- Reducing adverse drug reactions*

- Detecting genetic susceptibility to environmental carcinogens (which are linked to 50 to 95 percent of cancer risks)±

- Uncovering potential steroid hormone toxicity, which occurs in up to 40 percent of major population segments

- Optimizing drug and nutrient therapies to support healthy detoxification and overcome genetic predispositions to oxidative stress and disease

*If your body is not able to detoxify well, you may have an adverse drug reaction. Many health problems can be avoided and adverse reactions to medications and supplements can be prevented before they happen. For example, the Genovations test includes an evaluation of the gene CYP3A4, which affects an enzyme that your body uses to detoxify over 50 percent of all drugs. This can help prevent complications before they occur because if there is a problem with this system, you will be able to take care of it early on. These drugs include many antidepressants, steroid hormones (like estrogen), and cholesterol-lowering medications.

Adverse reactions to prescription drugs have been ranked anywhere from the fourth to the sixth leading cause of death in the United States. Each year about 100,000 Americans die from adverse reactions to medications—more than double the number of people killed in motor vehicle accidents. Annual hospital costs from these reactions have been estimated to be between $1 and $4 billion.

±The Genovations test also identifies increased genetic susceptibility to:

- Adverse drug reactions
- Fatigue syndromes
- Fibromyalgia
- Mood disorders
- Multiple chemical sensitivity
- Neurodegenerative disorders
- Numerous cancers
- Oxidative stress

**Detoxification and Nutrition**

You already learned that Phase I detoxification requires nutrients to be completed. In fact, the detoxification process as a whole is very nutrient-dependent. Phase I and Phase II enzymes are like the engines that drive the detoxification process, and they are fueled by vitamins, minerals, and other key food components. Therefore, if you are undernourished and lacking key vitamins or nutrients you may not be able to break down estrogen properly. This can leave estrogen available to cause cell transformation in the breasts and predispose you to breast cancer. Clearly, adequate nutrition is essential for effective detoxification.

- Increase in C-reactive protein (a marker of inflammation)
- Increase in gallstones
- Increase in sex hormone-binding globulin (SHBG), which can decrease testosterone
- Increase of estrone (E1)
- Increase of triglycerides
- Increased blood pressure
- Increased carbohydrate cravings
- Increased prothrombic effects (blood clots)
- Interruption in metabolism of tryptophan and serotonin, neurotransmitters that keep you calm and happy
- Weight gain

Estrogen creams are the preferred method of replacing this hormone that has so many functions. Many studies have been conducted on transdermal application of estradiol (E2). Transdermally applied, E2 has been shown to not impact liver synthesis of proteins the same way estrogen taken orally does. As stated in the list beginning on page 8, it also lowers triglycerides, which decreases your risk of heart disease. Finally, E2 applied to the skin does not negatively effect blood clotting.

When applied, it is important that you rub the estrogen in for two minutes. Discuss with your healthcare practitioner the best location on your skin to apply the estrogen, since it is best absorbed when applied to areas that contain fat cells—except for the abdomen.

## ESTROGEN AND YOUR BRAIN

Estrogen has many protective effects on your brain. One of these effects is that it acts as a natural antioxidant. Without optimal estrogen levels, you may find that your retrieval time for facts is not as quick, and your memory may decline. Common comments I hear from patients are: "I think that I am losing my mind," "I feel like my body is divorcing itself," "I have lost the ability to spell," "I am always losing my keys," and "I may be getting Alzheimer's disease."

## ■ Effects of Estrogen on the Brain

- Affects gene expression
- Boosts NMDA receptors by 30 percent in the brain to maintain strength and durability of synapse connections involved in creating long-term memories
- Decreases distractibility
- Decreases dopamine receptor sensitivity
- Decreases the risk of developing Alzheimer's disease
- Decreases the seizure threshold
- Enhances transmission of dopamine
- Improves the function of your neurons
- Increases availability of acetycholine, your neuro-transmitter of memory
- Increases availability of serotonin
- Increases blood flow
- Increases energy, mood, and feeling of well-being
- Increases excitability
- Increases GABA, a calming neurotransmitter
- Increases glucose and oxygen transportation to your neurons
- Increases manual speed and dexterity
- Increases norepinephrine effect, which gives you energy and helps you deal with stress
- Increases sensitivity to the nerve growth factor, which stimulates the growth of dendrites and axons in the brain
- Increases the production of choline acetyltransferase, which is needed for the production of acetylcholine, your main neurotransmitter of memory
- Increases verbal fluency and articulation
- Maintains the blood-brain barrier
- Protects neurons
- Regulates membrane channels
- Turns on progesterone receptors

Results from several studies have revealed that estrogen helps maintain your memory and cognitive function. It also increases your ability to learn new things. A Stanford University study showed that women who took estrogen were better able to recall people's names than women who did not take estrogen. Furthermore, a study done at McGill University in Canada found that women taking estrogen had better verbal memory than women who were not on hormone replacement therapy (HRT). (Verbal memory is when your brain and your mouth are connected—in other words, you do not forget words when you are speaking.)

Additionally, women on estrogen are less than half as likely to get Alzheimer's disease than women who are not on estrogen. Furthermore, estrogen use in post-menopausal women may delay the start of Alzheimer's.

A recent study conducted on 1,889 older women (at least sixty-five years old) in Utah revealed that the women who had taken HRT were 40 percent less likely to develop Alzheimer's disease. Furthermore, the longer the women were on HRT, the lower their risk was of developing the disease. (For a detailed description of HRT, see page 157.)

Estrogen does more than just help maintain memory. It is also a neuroactive hormone that reacts with receptors in your brain to modulate serotonin activity. A rapid change in estrogen levels can lead to decreased serotonin levels, which can cause depression.

In summary, estrogen has many protective effects on your brain, including maintaining your memory, decreasing the incidence of Alzheimer's disease, and lowering the rate of depression.

## PROGESTERONE

Progesterone is one of your sex hormones. It plays a role in menstruation, pregnancy, and the formation of embryos. Progesterone is made in the ovaries up until menopause. After menopause, it is made in the adrenal glands.

Progesterone performs many functions in your body aside from those listed above.

### ■ Functions of Progesterone in Your Body

- Balances estrogen

- Has a positive effect on your sleeping pattern

- Helps build bone

- Helps prevent anxiety, irritability, and mood swings

- Helps the bladder function

- Relaxes the smooth muscle in the gut so that your body can break down food into nutrients that are absorbed to be used elsewhere in the body

Sometimes, progesterone levels in the body drop below the optimal level. There are many reasons why this can happen (see the "Causes of Progesterone Deficiency" list below). When progesterone levels decline, there can be side effects, some more serious than others.

## ■ Symptoms of Progesterone Deficiency

☐ Anxiety

☐ Decreased HDL levels

☐ Decreased libido

☐ Depression

☐ Excessive menstruation (lasting longer than seven days and very heavy bleeding)

☐ Hypersensitivity

☐ Insomnia

☐ Irritability

☐ Migraine headaches prior to menstrual cycles

☐ Mood swings

☐ Nervousness

☐ Osteoporosis

☐ Pain and inflammation

☐ Weight gain

As mentioned, a progesterone deficiency can be caused by a variety of factors.

## ■ Causes of Progesterone Deficiency

• Antidepressants

• Decreased thyroid hormone

• Deficiency of vitamins A, $B_6$, C, and zinc

• Excessive arginine consumption

• Impaired production

• Increased prolactin production

• Low luteinizing hormone (LH)

• Saturated fat

• Stress

• Sugar

Just like your body can have too much estrogen, it can also have too much progesterone. Too much progesterone can have a variety of side effects.

## ■ Symptoms of Excess Progesterone

☐ Causes incontinence (leaky bladder)

☐ Causes ligaments to relax (can lead to backaches, leg aches, and achy hips)

- Decreases glucose tolerance (may predispose you to diabetes)
- Decreases growth hormone
- Increases appetite
- Increases carbohydrate cravings
- Increases cortisol
- Increases fat storage

- Increases insulin and insulin resistance
- Relaxes the smooth muscles of the gut (can cause bloating, fullness, and constipation; can also lead to gallstones)
- Suppresses the immune system

Unlike excess estrogen, which can be caused by a variety of factors, high progesterone levels can only result if a woman is taking too much progesterone or too much pregnenolone.

## NATURAL PROGESTERONE

Natural progesterone means that the progesterone that you are taking is the same chemical structure as the progesterone that you were born with. It is usually made from yams or soy. Synthetic progesterone, which will be discussed later in this section, is not the same chemical structure.

The process of producing natural progesterone was discovered by Russell Marker, a Pennsylvania State College chemistry professor. Back in the 1930s, Marker discovered that by using a chemical process, diosgenin (a plant steroid) could be turned into a form of progesterone that is an exact biological duplicate of the progesterone produced by the human body.

Natural progesterone, since it is biologically identical to the progesterone produced by the human body, has plenty of good effects not seen with synthetic progesterone. Consequently, many of these effects are similar to the effects of the progesterone that is produced by the body itself.

### ■ Effects of Natural Progesterone

- Balance estrogen levels
- Decreases the rate of cancer on all progesterone receptors
- Does not change the good effect estrogen has on blood flow
- Enhances the action of thyroid hormones
- Has a natural calming effect
- Balance fluids in the cells

- Helps restore proper cell oxygen levels
- Helps you sleep
- Helps your body use and eliminate fats
- Increases beneficial effects estrogen has on blood vessel dilation (hardened arteries)
- Increases metabolic rate
- Increases scalp hair
- Induces conversion of E1 to the inactive E1S form (E1S does not increase the risk of breast cancer)
- Is a natural antidepressant
- Is a natural diuretic (water pill)
- Is an anti-inflammatory
- Leaves the body quickly
- Lowers cholesterol
- Lowers high blood pressure
- May protect against breast cancer by inhibiting breast tissue overgrowth
- Normalizes and improves libido.
- Prevents migraine headaches that are menstrual cycle-related
- Promotes a healthy immune system
- Promotes myelination, which helps protect nerves from injury
- Relaxes smooth muscle
- Stimulates the production of new bone

## SYNTHETIC PROGESTERONE

Synthetic progesterone is called "progestin." It is very different from natural progesterone since it does not have the same chemical structure as the progesterone that your body makes on its own. Consequently, progestins do not reproduce the actions of natural progesterone (which have similar effects on the body as the progesterone the body produces itself). For example, progestins do not help balance the estrogen in the body. They interfere with the body's production of its own progesterone, and when they're in your body, they attach to many of your body's receptor sites, not just the progesterone receptors. Furthermore, progestins stop the protective effects estrogen has on your heart, and can cause spasms of your arteries.

A recent study has shown that the use of synthetic progesterone increases the risk of breast cancer by 800 percent when compared to the use of estrogen alone. An article in the *Journal of the American Medical Association* discussed that the risk of developing breast cancer was predicted to rise by nearly 80 percent after ten years of using estrogen and/or progestin (synthetic) HRT.

Likewise, Dr. Stephen Sinatra, a well-known cardiologist, states in his book *Heart Sense for Women*, "I have found that synthetic progestins can lead to serious cardiac side effects in my patients, including shortness of breath, fatigue, chest pain, and high blood pressure."

Progestins may have other side effects that do not occur with natural progesterone.

## ■ Side Effects of Progestins

- Acne
- Bloating
- Breakthrough bleeding/spotting
- Breast tenderness
- Counteracts many of the positive effects estrogen has on serotonin
- Decrease in energy
- Decrease in sexual interest
- Decreased HDL (good cholesterol)
- Depression
- Fluid retention
- Hair loss
- Headaches
- Inability to help produce estrogen and testosterone
- Increased appetite
- Increased LDL (bad cholesterol)
- Insomnia
- Irritability
- Nausea
- Protects only the uterus from cancer (not the breasts)
- Rashes
- Remains in your body longer than natural progesterone, which can prevent it from balancing with the other hormones
- Weight gain

There are, however, a few positive effects of progestins, all of which are also effects of natural progesterone. For example, both build bone, help the thyroid hormone function, protect against fibrocystic breast disease and endometrial cancer, and normalize zinc and copper levels.

Aside from these few common positive effects, it is clear from this discussion that natural progesterone offers a safer approach to HRT than synthetic progesterone (progestin) does. It is also very important that you have your levels of progesterone measured before you begin HRT, and then on a regular basis afterwards to confirm that you are taking an optimal dose for you. (See the section on testing on page 161.)

Progesterone can be taken orally or used transdermally. After receiving your prescription, you'll need a compounding pharmacist in order to get it filled. As mentioned, natural progesterone is made from yams or soy. Your compounding pharmacist will add an enzyme to convert the hormone from these plants (disogenin) into progesterone. Over-the-counter progesterone, which you can buy without a prescription, frequently does not contain this enzyme.

If you're suffering from insomnia and you need to take progesterone, you should opt for the pill form. The pill affects the GABA receptors in your brain. GABA is an amino acid that acts as a neurotransmitter. It has a calming effect on your brain, which helps you sleep.

Natural progesterone is also available as Prometrium, which is a pill derived from peanut oil made by a pharmaceutical company. The absorption rate of oral progesterone increases as you age, so you need less medication as you grow older. As women age, progesterone applied transdermally is commonly used. Some women experience side effects from oral progesterone, such as nausea, breast swelling, dizziness, drowsiness, and depression, due to its effects on the liver and gastrointestinal tract.

Many women who have had a complete hysterectomy wonder if they still need progesterone. The answer is yes. Natural progesterone has many positive effects on the body, as previously discussed.

Lastly, adrenaline also interacts with progesterone. When a person feels stressed, his or her adrenaline surges, which can block progesterone receptors. This can prevent progesterone from being used effectively in the body.

## ESTROGEN/PROGESTERONE RATIO

You've already learned about estrogen and progesterone. But did you know that it is important that the two hormones remain in a specific ratio within your body?

As you will learn, there is an increased risk of breast cancer if estrogen metabolism favors the 16-hydroxyestrone pathway. There is also a higher risk for breast cancer if you have a low progesterone-to-estrogen ratio, which means that the estrogen and progesterone ratio in your body is out of balance.

Having a low progesterone-to-estrogen ratio can have other effects on the body as well.

## ■ Effects of a Low Progesterone-to-Estrogen Ratio

- Abnormal bleeding during peri- and postmenopause
- Increased risk of breast cancer
- Increased risk of uterine cancer
- Infertility

Estrogen and progesterone work together in your body. E2 (one of the forms of estrogen your body makes) lowers body fat by decreasing the amount of lipoprotein lipase, an enzyme, in your fat cells. Progesterone increases body fat storage by increasing the amount of lipoprotein lipase.

Estrogen and progesterone also work together to balance your body's release of insulin. E2 increases insulin sensitivity and improves glucose tolerance. Progesterone decreases insulin sensitivity and can cause insulin resistance. For this reason, women who have diabetes need to make sure that their estrogen/progesterone ratio is normal.

An estrogen/progesterone ratio that is too high in progesterone will break down protein and muscle tissue, which will make diseases (like fibromyalgia, an autoimmune disease that causes muscle pain) worse.

There are other side effects of a high progesterone-to-estrogen ratio.

## ■ Effects of a High Progesterone-to-Estrogen Ratio

- Decrease in sexual interest
- Depression
- Fatigue
- Insulin resistance/diabetes

If you use progesterone for too long without adequately using estrogen, there can be negative side effects.

## ■ Side Effects of Progesterone Without Adequate Estrogen Use*

- Decreased HDL (good cholesterol)
- Decreased libido
- Depression
- Fatigue
- Increased insulin resistance (can predispose you to diabetes)
- Increased LDL (bad cholesterol)
- Increased total cholesterol
- Increased triglyceride levels
- Weight gain

*See the list on page 7 to learn what can happen if you have too much estrogen and not enough progesterone.*

When you have a salivary test or a twenty-four-hour urine test done to measure your hormone levels, your healthcare practitioner will also get a measure of the estrogen/progesterone ratio. He or she will then prescribe the appropriate treatment according to the lab results.

# TESTOSTERONE

Testosterone falls into a class of hormones called "androgens." Androgens are commonly referred to as "male" hormones, but they are present in women as well. The reason they are called male is because the human characteristics they stimulate and control are considered to be masculine characteristics.

Testosterone is made in the adrenal glands and ovaries. For most women as they age, the ovaries produce less testosterone. Of this testosterone, only one percent is free, meaning it is available for the body to use. The rest is bound to sex-hormone binding globulin (SHGB).

Women who have increased levels of androgens have higher levels of free testosterone. Therefore, it is important for these women to measure their salivary or urinary hormone levels and not just their blood hormone levels (see page 161 for salivary testing). This is important since your hormone levels flux throughout your cycle. Also, salivary or urinary hormone levels are a measure of the hormones in your entire body and not just the levels in your blood.

Testosterone performs many important functions in the body.

## ■ Functions of Testosterone in Your Body

- Decreases bone deterioration
- Decreases excess body fat
- Elevates norepinephrine in the brain (has the same effect as taking an antidepressant)
- Helps maintain memory
- Increases muscle mass and strength
- Increases muscle tone (so your skin doesn't sag)
- Increases sense of emotional well-being, self-confidence, and motivation
- Increases sexual interest (86 percent of woman say they experience a decrease in sexual interest with menopause)

Women of any age can experience a deficiency of testosterone, which is indicated by a variety of symptoms.

## ■ Symptoms of Testosterone Deficiency

☐ Anxiety

☐ Decline in muscle tone

☐ Decreased HDL (good cholesterol)

☐ Decreased sex drive

☐ Droopy eyelids

☐ Dry, thin skin with poor elasticity

☐ Dry, thinning hair

☐ Fatigue

☐ Hypersensitive, hyperemotional states

☐ Less dreaming

☐ Loss of pubic hair

☐ Low self-esteem

☐ Mild depression

☐ Muscle wasting (despite adequate calorie and protein intake)

☐ Saggy cheeks

☐ Thin lips

☐ Weight gain

## ■ Causes of Testosterone Deficiency

• Adrenal stress or burnout

• Birth control pills, which increase SHBG (see page 167)

• Chemotherapy

• Childbirth

• Cholesterol-lowering medications

• Depression

• Endometriosis

• Menopause

• Psychological trauma

• Surgical menopause

## ■ Ways to Increase Testosterone Levels

• Decrease your calorie intake

• Exercise

• Get enough sleep (at least seven hours a night is an adequate amount)

• Increase the amount of protein in your diet

• Lose weight

• Practice stress reduction

• Take arginine, leucine, or glutamine (amino acids)

• Take zinc, which helps metabolize testosterone

Like other hormones, you can have too much testosterone in your body. Excess production of androgens is usually due to over-production by your adrenal glands, but this can also be from your ovaries. Androgen dominance is the most common hormonal disorder in women. Almost 10 percent of all women have had or will have some kind of androgen imbalance in their lifetime. In younger woman, adrenal imbalance is commonly related to PCOS (see page 122). As women go through menopause, about 20 percent of them will experience high testosterone levels that will not decline with age.

## ■ Symptoms of Excess Testosterone

☐ Acne or oily skin

☐ Agitation

☐ Anger

☐ Anxiety

☐ Changes in memory

☐ Decreased HDL (good cholesterol)

☐ Depression

☐ Fatigue

☐ Fluid retention

☐ Hair loss

☐ Hirsutism (facial hair)

☐ Hypoglycemia

☐ Increased insulin resistance

☐ Increased risk of developing breast cancer

☐ Infertility

☐ Irregular periods

☐ Mood swings

☐ Poor prognosis if you have breast cancer

☐ Salt and sugar cravings

☐ Weight gain

There are some things you can do to lower your testosterone levels. You can take saw palmetto (an herb), glucophage (a prescription), or spironolactone (a prescription). However, reduction of testosterone should be done only under the guidance of a healthcare professional.

As you can see, replacement of testosterone and regulation of the amount of testosterone in your body throughout your life are required for you to have optimal health.

Dihydrotestosterone (DHT) is a byproduct of testosterone. High DHT levels can cause hair loss in women. You can have your DHT levels measured by taking a blood test. In the body, DHT makes androstanediol, another androgen. Androstanediol levels can be measured with a urine sample (see section on urine tests, page 162). Elevated urinary androstanediol has been observed in people who have PCOS, hirsutism, visceral obesity, and post-menopausal women who have breast cancer.

5-alpha-reductase is an enzyme that is present in the conversion of testosterone to androstanediol. High levels of 5-alpha-reductase are associated with insulin resistance, obesity, high-protein diets, sodium (salt) restriction, licorice (a supplement or a food), hyperthyroidism (high thyroid levels), and DHEA supplementation. Lower levels of this enzyme are seen in vegetarians, people who use progesterone, epigallocatechin gallate (EGCG, which is in green tea), flaxseed ligans, medications such as *Proscar* and *Propecia*, and the intake of saw palmetto, pygeum, and stinging nettles.

SHBG is a carrier protein for testosterone and DHT, and somewhat for estradiol (E2). If SHBG levels are high, there is less E2 and testosterone available for use by the body. Likewise, low SHBG levels mean there is more E2 and testosterone available for use. Low SHBG levels may be a marker for low thyroid function. High insulin levels and high prolactin levels change the levels of SHBG.

If you are taking estrogen orally, it can increase your SHBG by 50 percent. If you are taking Premarin, your SHBG levels can increase by 100 percent. Transdermally-applied estrogen nominally increases SHBG, unless you overdose.

## TESTOSTERONE AND ESTROGEN

Research shows that in order for testosterone to work well, E2 must also be optimized. Without enough estrogen present, testosterone cannot attach to your brain receptors. Therefore, estrogen plays a role in how well testosterone works in your body.

If testosterone is taken with E2, it lowers your cardiac risk. If your estrogen levels are low and you take testosterone alone, it can increase plaque formation in your heart vessels, which increases your risk of having a heart attack.

## NATURAL AND SYNTHETIC TESTOSTERONE

Natural testosterone is the preferred method of testosterone replacement. Synthetic testosterone, or methyltestosterone, has been associated with an increased risk of liver cancer.

Natural testosterone is effective when taken as a pill or applied as a cream, but it is more commonly used as a cream. However, if you are using it as a cream, remember to rotate application sites. Applying the cream to the same location all the time will result in an increase in hair growth in that section. Unfortunately, this does not work to re-grow hair on your head.

# DHEA

DHEA is another one of your sex hormones. It is made by your adrenal glands, but a small amount is also made in your brain and skin. DHEA production declines with age, starting in the late twenties. By the age of seventy, your body only makes one-fourth of the amount it made earlier. DHEA also makes your estrogen and testosterone.

## ■ Functions of DHEA in Your Body

- Decreases allergic reactions
- Decreases cholesterol
- Decreases formation of fatty deposits
- Helps you deal with stress
- Helps your body repair itself and maintain tissues
- Increases bone growth
- Increases brain function
- Increases lean body mass
- Increases sense of well-being
- Lowers triglycerides
- Prevents blood clots
- Promotes weight loss
- Reduces insulin resistance
- Reduces spikes in blood sugar
- Supports your immune system

Low DHEA levels can occur at any age.

## ■ Symptoms of DHEA Deficiency

- ☐ Decreased energy
- ☐ Decreased muscle strength
- ☐ Difficulty dealing with stress
- ☐ Increased risk of infection
- ☐ Irritability
- ☐ Joint soreness
- ☐ Weight gain

There are many things that can contribute to a DHEA deficiency. Women are more sensitive to the effects of DHEA than men, and therefore they need less DHEA than men do.

## ■ Causes of DHEA Deficiency

- Aging
- Decreased production
- Menopause
- Smoking (nicotine inhibits the production of 11-beta-hydroxylase, an enzyme needed to make DHEA)
- Stress

If your body has a low DHEA level, it would be a good idea to consider DHEA replacement. There are many benefits of replacing DHEA, which can be supplemented orally or with a cream. For example, DHEA has been shown to have a protective effect against cancer, diabetes, obesity, high cholesterol, heart disease, and autoimmune diseases.

### ◼ Benefits of Replacing DHEA

- Activates immune system function
- Decreases joint stiffness
- Elevates growth hormone levels
- Improves sleep
- Increases feeling of well-being
- Increases muscle strength and lean body mass
- Increases quality of life (you'll have more energy, less infections, an improved mood, etc.)
- Increases sensitivity of insulin (helps sugar levels stay normal)

Studies conducted at the University of Tennessee revealed that supplementing with DHEA produced a 30 percent reduction in insulin levels when compared to taking the diabetes drug, *Metformin*, alone. Importantly, the supplements also tripled patients' sensitivity to insulin. This result may be due to the fact that diabetics may have lower levels of DHEA in their bodies then people who have normal blood sugar levels.

However, like most other hormones, you can overdose and have too much DHEA in your body.

### ◼ Symptoms of Excess DHEA

- ☐ Acne
- ☐ Anger
- ☐ Deeper voice
- ☐ Depression
- ☐ Facial hair
- ☐ Fatigue
- ☐ Insomnia
- ☐ Irritability
- ☐ Mood changes
- ☐ Restless sleep
- ☐ Sugar cravings
- ☐ Weight gain

### ◼ Causes of Excess DHEA

- Stress
- Taking too much DHEA
- Tumor in the adrenal glands

# CORTISOL

Cortisol is the only hormone in your body that increases with age. It is also one of your sex hormones. Like DHEA, cortisol is made by your adrenal glands, which make all your sex hormones after menopause. Cortisol is commonly known as the "stress hormone" due to its involvement in your response to stress.

## ■ Functions of Cortisol in Your Body

- Affects bone turnover rate
- Affects immune system response
- Affects pituitary/thyroid/adrenal system
- Affects stress reaction
- Balances blood sugar
- Controls weight
- Helps protein synthesis
- Helps you sleep
- Improves mood and thoughts
- Influences DHEA/insulin ratio
- Influences estrogen/testosterone ratio
- Is an anti-inflammatory
- Participates with aldosterone in sodium reabsorption

When you are stressed, your cortisol levels elevate. (The relationship between cortisol and stress will be discussed later in this section.)

However, there are also consequences of low cortisol levels. When your adrenal glands are in a state of emergency, you do not feel well. You may turn to coffee, soft drinks, or sugar as a source of energy, but this will only make the situation worse. Consuming any of these items will temporarily make you feel better or more energetic, but the negative effects far outweigh the temporary fix. If your adrenal glands stay stimulated when they are in a state of emergency, they may weaken and "burn out." When this happens, your cortisol and DHEA levels will drop. This is called adrenal fatigue.

If the adrenals become totally depleted, it is called Addison's disease. This is a medical emergency. If you have Addison's disease, your body makes no cortisol at all. Adrenal fatigue is not a total depletion of cortisol, but it does bring cortisol levels down low enough to prevent optimal functioning of the body. Adrenal fatigue is one of the most pervasive and under-diagnosed syndromes of modern society. (A deficiency of cortisol that is not Addison's disease is usually caused by stress.)

## ■ Symptoms of Adrenal Fatigue (Cortisol Deficiency)

☐ Alcoholism

☐ Allergies (environmental sensitivities and chemical intolerance)

☐ Decreased immunity

☐ Decreased sexual interest

☐ Digestive problems

☐ Drug addiction

☐ Emotional imbalances

☐ Emotional paralysis

☐ Fatigue

☐ Feeling of being overwhelmed

☐ General feeling of "unwellness"

☐ Hypoglycemia (low blood sugar)

☐ Increased PMS, perimenopausal, and menopausal symptoms

☐ Lack of stamina

☐ Loss of motivation or initiative

☐ Low blood pressure

☐ Poor healing of wounds

☐ Progressively poorer athletic performance

☐ Sensitivity to light

☐ Unresponsive hypothyroidism (low thyroid function that doesn't respond to treatment)

Abnormal cortisol levels that are too high or too low can be associated with many medical conditions.

## ■ Conditions Associated With Abnormal Levels of Cortisol

- Alzheimer's disease
- Anorexia nervosa
- Breast cancer
- Chronic fatigue syndrome
- Coronary heart disease
- Depression
- Diabetes
- Exacerbations of multiple sclerosis
- Fibromyalgia
- Generalized memory loss
- Heart disease
- Impotence
- Infertility
- Insulin resistance
- Irritable bowel syndrome (IBS)
- Menopause
- Osteoporosis
- Panic disorders
- PMS
- Post-traumatic stress disorder (PTSD)
- Rheumatiod arthritis
- Sleep disorders

Many women enter menopause with a less-than-adequate amount of progesterone due to an exhaustion of their adrenal glands. If you are experiencing a burnout, your doctor can treat you with DHEA. Or, if all other treatments fail, low dose cortef may help do the trick. Be sure to have your levels measured before you start on any of these hormones. In my practice, I also recommend some herbs for this purpose, such as Cordyceps (Cordyceps sinensis), Asian ginseng (Panax ginseng), and Rhodiola (Rhodiola rosea).

Licorice root, an herbal supplement made from the licorice plant, decreases the amount of hydrocortisone that is broken down by the liver, which reduces the demand on the adrenals to produce more cortisol. Licorice root can raise your blood pressure, so it should not be taken if you have hypertension. Additionally, adrenal extracts, which are made from the adrenal glands of animals and are purified, can also be used to elevate cortisol levels.

There are also nutrients that help support adrenal function.

### ■ Nutrients Associated With Increasing Adrenal Function

- B-vitamins
- Calcium
- Copper
- Magnesium
- Manganese
- Omega-3-fatty acids, such as fish oil
- Phosphatidylserine
- Selenium
- Sodium
- Vitamin C
- Zinc

Usually, it takes six months of constant stress or more for adrenal fatigue to settle in. However, once you start treatment for your exhausted adrenals, it takes one to two years for your glands to heal completely.

There are other things you can do to help treat adrenal fatigue. Restful sleep (sleeping until 9 AM or later), resolving a stressful situation, lying down during a break from work, going to bed early (around 9 PM), and avoiding eating fruit in the morning can all help. Clearly, trying these options before things get out of hand is a good idea. If adrenal fatigue can be helped or improved, the overall healing time will be shortened.

Many women who have adrenal fatigue also have a thyroid that isn't functioning to its full potential (hypothyroidism). It is important to always work on fixing the adrenal glands before thyroid medication is instituted; otherwise, the symptoms of adrenal fatigue may be made worse.

Adrenal fatigue is a symptom that can dramatically affect your health and can be reversed with proper treatment. Lifestyle changes, good nutrition, dietary supplements, and stress reduction techniques have all proven to be affective.

## CORTISOL AND STRESS

When you are stressed, cortisol levels elevate. As stress decreases, levels come back down. However, in today's world, a lot of people are stressed a lot of the time. Overbooking is an issue with almost everyone. If you have too many tasks on your plate or you multitask all of the time, your body will remain in a state of constant stress.

The most important thing you can do to get rid of your stress is to gain control of your time. Learn to say "no" kindly. Know how much work and responsibility you can take on without feeling overwhelmed, and do not take on more than you can handle. It is also useful to practice some relaxing techniques that you can turn to in times of stress. Running a hot bath, drinking a cup of coffee or tea, listening to your favorite song, or curling up with a good book are all effective ways to reduce stress. Figure out what works for you, and turn to it if you feel your stress levels rising.

Carl Sandberg, a famous American poet, once wrote:

*Time is the coin of your life. It is the only coin you have,*
*and only you can determine how it will be spent.*
*Be careful lest you let other people spend it for you.*

Stress can be harnessed to fuel success and achievement. However, if your stress is to the point of "distress," then that is a problem. Magnesium, potassium, B-vitamins, vitamin C, zinc, carbohydrates, and other nutrients are used up when you are stressed.

Your brain is one of the body parts that is most affected by stress. When you are stressed and your cortisol levels increase, your body produces more free radicals. This damages your neurons and decreases your ability to think and remember things. When this happens, your body's ability to change short-term memories into long-term memories is affected. Your ability to recall and retrieve information is also affected by stress. High levels of cortisol are associated with deterioration of the hippocampus, the part of your brain that processes memory.

# Other Signs of Stress

By this point, you have learned that stress greatly affects cortisol levels, causing them to elevate. Elevated cortisol levels can have many negative consequences, which can be seen in the list starting at the bottom of this page.

Over the years, I have compiled a list of common signs of stress, which can be divided into four categories.

Behavioral symptoms can be seen in the way you act. Some behavioral symptoms include bossiness, compulsive eating or gum chewing, excessive smoking, grinding your teeth at night, alcohol abuse, and an inability to focus and complete tasks.

Cognitive symptoms are those that affect the way you think. If you are stressed, you may experience constant worry, forgetfulness, memory loss, or a lack of creativity. Additionally, you may have difficulty making decisions, lose your sense of humor, or have thoughts of running away.

Emotional symptoms affect your mood and feelings. If you're stressed, you may find that you are easily upset. Additionally, you may experience a range of emotions, including anger, boredom, edginess, loneliness, nervousness, anxiety, and unhappiness. Finally, people who are stressed commonly feel like they are under pressure, and they often feel powerless to change anything.

Lastly, there are some physical symptoms of stress that affect your body. These include back pain, dizziness, headaches, a racing heart, restlessness, indigestion, stomachaches, tiredness, sweaty palms, a stiff neck or shoulders, ringing in the ears, and difficulty sleeping.

If you find that you are experiencing any of these symptoms, it would be a good idea to try and lower your levels of stress (some suggestions for how you can do this are on page 35). You will benefit in the long run.

In addition to stress, cortisol levels also increase with depression, high progestin intake, birth control pills, infections, inadequate sleep, inflammation, hypoglycemia (low blood sugar), toxic exposure, and pain.

## ■ Long-Term Consequences of Elevated Cortisol

- Binge eating
- Confusion
- Fatigue
- Impaired hepatic conversion of T4 to T3 (see thyroid section, page 43)

- Increased blood pressure
- Increased blood sugar
- Increased cholesterol
- Increased insulin and insulin resistance

- Increased risk of developing osteoporosis
- Increased susceptibility to bruising
- Increased susceptibility to infections
- Increased triglycerides
- Irritability
- Low energy
- Night sweats
- Shakiness between meals
- Sleep disturbances
- Sugar cravings
- Thinning skin
- Weakened muscles
- Weakened immune system the middle)

All of the hormones in your body work together—they are a symphony. In order for you to have good health, they all have to be balanced and at optimal levels. If your cortisol levels are increased, your body's production of progesterone decreases. Cortisol competes with progesterone for common receptors. When cortisol levels are elevated, the thyroid gland is directly affected. The thyroid hormone that is produced may become stored, or bound, in the body, and therefore it will be unavailable for your body to use.

Having decreased levels of estradiol (E2) is also a stressor on your body because it causes cortisol levels to rise. Decreased E2 also causes a decrease in optimal function of norepinephrine, serotonin, dopamine, and acetylcholine, which are your neurotransmitters responsible for communication between your cells.

## ■ Factors Regulated by Neurotransmitters

- Appetite
- Memory
- Mood
- Muscle growth and repair
- Sexual interest
- Sleep
- Thirst
- Weight

The simplest way to stop your cortisol levels from increasing is to better manage your stress. However, as you get older, this becomes more difficult because your ability to bounce back after a stressful event is reduced. Each event takes a deeper and more lasting toll on your body. Premature aging and many age-related disorders can begin with excessive stress.

Of course, abnormal levels of cortisol can occur at any age, but there are certainly different factors that can affect stress levels. One such factor is your job. Some jobs create more stress than others.

## ■ Most Stressful Occupations According to the National Institutes of Health

- Construction worker
- Farm worker
- Foreman/supervisor
- House painter
- Laboratory technician
- Machine operator
- Midlevel manager
- Secretary
- Waiter or waitress

The jobs on the list have one thing in common: a lack of control. Remember, you may not be able to control the things that are stressing you, but you can control how you respond to the stress. In other words, the key is not to avoid stress, but to change your perspective and how you respond to stress.

Stress reduction techniques are a key component to healing. Prayer, meditation, tai chi (a Chinese form of martial arts), yoga, chi gong (a form of body and mind therapy), breathing exercises and techniques, exercise (not strenuous exercise if you have adrenal fatigue), music, and dancing have all been shown to be therapeutic.

In order to be healthy, you have to be physically healthy, emotionally healthy, and spiritually healthy. All of these areas of your life have to be optimally functioning in order for you to be stress-free.

# PREGNENOLONE

Pregnenolone is a steroid hormone. It is a precursor to (makes) DHEA, progesterone, estrogen, testosterone, and cortisol. Your body synthesizes this hormone from cholesterol.

Pregnenolone levels decrease with age. By age seventy-five, you have 65 percent less pregnenolone than you do at age thirty-five. It is rare that someone in their twenties or thirties would need this hormone.

In addition to making many of your other hormones, pregnenolone has a variety of other functions.

## ■ Functions of Pregnenolone in Your Body

- Blocks the production of acid-forming compounds
- Enhances nerve transmission and memory
- Helps to repair nerve damage
- Improves energy (physically and mentally)
- Improves sleep

- Increases resistance to stress
- Modulates the neurotransmitter GABA
- Modulates NMDA receptors (regulates pain control, learning, memory, and alertness)
- Promotes mood elevation
- Reduces pain and inflammation
- Regulates the balance between excitation and inhibition in the nervous system

Your natural pathways of pregnenolone are blocked when you eat too much saturated fat and trans-fatty acids. When this occurs, you do not make the optimum amounts of your other sex hormones. Also, when you have a severe illness, such as diabetes, pregnenolone makes more cortisol and less of the other hormones to help you deal with the stress. You can see how important it is for your body's hormonal symphony to be playing in tune.

## ■ Symptoms of Pregnenolone Deficiency

- ☐ Arthritis
- ☐ Depression
- ☐ Fatigue
- ☐ Inability to deal with stress
- ☐ Insomnia
- ☐ Lack of focus
- ☐ Memory decline

The only known causes of pregnenolone deficiency are the aging process, low cholesterol levels, hypothyroidism, and a pituitary tumor.

Like any other hormone, you can overuse pregnenolone. Therefore, it is important to have your pregnenolone levels measured by a fellowship-trained Metabolic/Anti-Aging specialist before you begin supplementation. Pregnenolone makes the other sex hormones, and therefore should not be used unless you have your levels measured, since it can lead to an imbalance of your other sex hormones.

## ■ Symptoms of Excess Pregnenolone

- ☐ Acne
- ☐ Drowsiness
- ☐ Fluid retention
- ☐ Headache
- ☐ Heart racing (palpatations)
- ☐ Insomnia due to overstimulation
- ☐ Irritability, anger, anxiety
- ☐ Muscle aches

Pregnenolone can be applied as a cream or taken by mouth. Studies that date back to the 1960s have shown that pregnenolone used as a cream had positive effects on the skin. Researchers noted that at the end of three months, the participants' skin was more hydrated, had fewer wrinkles, and appeared fuller.

Pregnenolone is also used for the treatment of arthritis, depression, memory loss, fatigue, and moodiness. Supplementation with pregnenolone has also been found to be useful in treating autoimmune diseases such as rheumatoid arthritis, ankylosing spondylitis, and lupus. Furthermore, the use of pregnenolone with other sex hormones (such as estrogen, progesterone, testosterone, or DHEA) allows for smaller doses of these hormones to be used and is less physiologically disturbing.

Pregnenolone has also been shown to improve delta-wave sleep, the deep, dreamless stage of sleeping. As you age, the amount of delta-wave sleep that you get declines. This lowers melatonin levels and growth hormone production and can lead to premature aging. People with hypothyroidism have been shown, in some studies, to also have low pregnenolone levels. This is part of the hormonal symphony. All the musicians must play in tune in order for you to have optimal results.

## INSULIN

Your body makes a hormone called insulin to help you regulate your blood sugar.

### ■ Functions of Insulin in Your Body

- Counters the actions of adrenaline and cortisol in the body
- Helps the body repair
- Helps to convert blood sugar into triglycerides
- Keeps blood glucose levels from rising too high
- Plays a major role in the production of serotonin (your "happy" neurotransmitter)
- Stimulates the development of muscle, but at high levels it turns off the production of muscle and increases the production of fat

You do not want your insulin levels to be too low, which can result in insulin not working as well as it should. If your insulin levels are too low, you may experience some negative symptoms.

## ■ Symptoms of Insulin Deficiency

☐ Bone Loss                    ☐ Fatigue

☐ Depression                   ☐ Insomnia

## ■ Causes of Insulin Deficiency

- Eliminating carbohydrates from       • Not eating enough
  your diet                            • Over-exercising

When you eat complex carbohydrates and simple sugars, your insulin levels climb. If you eat too much sugar, your body produces more and more insulin until the insulin does not work as effectively as it should. The medical term for this is "insulin resistance," but I like to call it "insulin impotence."

## ■ Symptoms of Excess Insulin

☐ Acne                            ☐ High blood pressure

☐ Aging process accelerates       ☐ High cholesterol

☐ Asthma                          ☐ High triglycerides

☐ Breast cancer                   ☐ Infertility

☐ Colon cancer                    ☐ Insomnia

☐ Depression and mood swings      ☐ Irritable bowel syndrome

☐ Estrogen levels that are too low ☐ Migraine headaches

☐ Heart disease                   ☐ Osteopenia/osteoporosis

☐ Heartburn                       ☐ Weight gain

Insulin is part of the hormonal symphony in your body so when it is not doing its job well, all the other hormones are affected. Your body will attempt to compensate for insulin's decreased effect by producing more and more insulin. This can result in high insulin levels all of the time, which can cause the cells in your adrenal glands, called theca cells, to turn on an enzyme called 17, 20-lyase. 17, 20-lyase causes your body's hormones to stop making estrogens and instead make androgens. (Both estrogens and androgens are made from DHEA.) This shift in hormonal balance can cause you to gain weight around the middle. It may also promote further insulin resistance. In fact, prolonged levels of high insulin can lead to diabetes. Furthermore, every major process that leads to "hardening of the arteries" is caused by the overproduction of insulin.

When you eat simple sugars and intake caffeine to help with fatigue, not only will your adrenal glands suffer, but this will contribute to an elevated level of insulin in your body. Additionally, this causes your body to produce gas and you may experience bloating. Water is pulled into your colon from the bloodstream to respond to the high sugar load, which can lead to loose stools. If you overeat carbohydrates you can develop a sensitivity to gluten, which is in wheat products.

There are many habits that can elevate insulin levels besides eating a diet high in simple sugars. The following list contains lifestyle choices that raise insulin, as per Dr. Diana Schwarzbein, an endocrinologist and author of *The Schwarzbein Principle* and *The Schwarzbein Principle II*.

### ■ Causes of Excess Insulin Production

- Consuming soft drinks
- Diet pills
- Eating a low-fat diet
- Eating trans-fats (partially-hydrogenated or hydrogenated foods)
- Elevated DHEA levels
- Excessive alcohol consumption
- Excess caffeine intake
- Excessive or unnecessary thyroid hormone medication
- Excessive progesterone replacement
- Increased testosterone levels
- Insomnia
- Lack of exercise
- Low estrogen levels
- Skipping meals

- Smoking
- Some over-the-counter cold medications (any that contain caffeine)
- Some prescription medications:
  Beta-blockers
  Birth control pills
  Some medications for depression and psychosis
  Steriods
  Thiazide diuretics (water pills)
- Stress
- Taking hypothyroid medication while not eating enough
- Use of natural stimulants
- Use of recreational stimulants
- Using artificial sweeteners
- Yo-yo dieting

Elevated insulin levels can be lowered by eating a balanced diet of carbohydrates, proteins, and fats. The right amount of exercise (three to four times a week) can normalize insulin levels. Changing medications, quitting smoking, discontinuing stimulants, and stopping caffeine consumption can also be helpful.

There are also nutrients that can help insulin work more effectively in the body. Alpha lipoic acid, chromium, and vitamin D all do just this. However, these supplements can be very powerful, so if you are already taking a drug that lowers your blood sugar you may need less medication with the use of these products. Make sure you monitor your blood sugar closely. Alpha lipoic acid has even been used to prevent and treat diabetic neuropathy, a condition where the body's nerves become damaged due to diabetes.

# THYROID HORMONE

Your thyroid gland is your body regulator. Therefore, an imbalance of your thyroid hormone can affect every metabolic function in your body.

Your thyroid gland has a lot of important functions.

### ■ Functions of the Thyroid Gland and Thyroid Hormone in Your Body

- Affects tissue repair and development
- Aides in the function of mitochondria (energy makers of your cells)
- Assists in the digestion process
- Controls hormone excretion
- Controls oxygen utilization
- Modulates blood flow
- Modulates carbohydrate, protein, and fat metabolism
- Modulates muscle and nerve action
- Modulates sexual function
- Regulates energy and heat production
- Regulates growth
- Regulates vitamin usage
- Stimulates protein synthesis

## TYPES OF THYROID HORMONE

It is common for thyroid problems to appear at menopause. Your ovaries have thyroid receptors, and your thyroid gland has ovarian receptors. Therefore, the loss of estradiol (E2) and testosterone from your ovaries that occurs at menopause can have an effect on your thyroid.

There are a few different types of thyroid hormones that your body produces. They are:

- Diiodothyronine (T2)

- Thyroid stimulating hormone (TSH), which is made in your pituitary gland located in your brain

- Thyroxine (T4), which is made in your thyroid gland

- Triiodothyronine (T3), which is made in other tissues

T4 is 80 percent of the thyroid gland's production. Most of T4 is converted into T3 in your liver or kidneys. T3 is five times more active than T4.

T4 can also be converted into reverse T3, which is an inactive (stored) form. Taking too much T4 is the most common reason for this.

Additionally, T2 increases the metabolic rate of your muscles and fat tissues.

## HYPOTHYROIDISM (LOW THYROID FUNCTION)

Since your thyroid is important to so many functions in your body, it may seem natural that many side effects could result if your thyroid levels aren't at their optimal amounts.

### ■ Symptoms of Low Thyroid Production (Hypothyroidism)

☐ Agitation

☐ Allergies

☐ Anxiety/panic attacks

☐ Arrhythmias (irregular heart rhythm)

☐ Brittle nails

☐ Carpal tunnel syndrome

☐ Coarse, dry hair

☐ Cold hands and feet

☐ Constipation

☐ Decreased cardiac output

☐ Decreased memory

☐ Decreased sexual interest

☐ Deposition of mucin in connective tissues (this helps the tissues move well)

☐ Depression

☐ Diffuse hair loss

☐ Dizziness/vertigo

☐ Down-turned mouth

☐ Drooping eyelids

☐ Dry, itchy ear canals

☐ Dull facial expression

☐ Elbow keratosis

☐ Endometriosis

☐ Excess formation of cerumen (ear wax)

- [ ] Fat buildup at the clavicle (collar bone)
- [ ] Fatigue
- [ ] Fibrocystic breast disease (noncancerous changes in the breast tissues)
- [ ] Fluid retention
- [ ] Gallstones
- [ ] Headaches
- [ ] High blood pressure
- [ ] High cholesterol
- [ ] High insulin levels
- [ ] Hoarse, husky voice
- [ ] Hypoglycemia (low blood sugar)
- [ ] Inability to concentrate
- [ ] Increase in blepharospasm (eye spasm)
- [ ] Increased appetite
- [ ] Increased risk of developing asthma
- [ ] Increased susceptibility to bruising
- [ ] Infertility
- [ ] Insomnia
- [ ] Intolerance to cold temperatures
- [ ] Iron deficiency anemia
- [ ] Irregularities in menstrual cycle
- [ ] Joint pain or stiffness
- [ ] Loss of hair (varying amounts) from legs, arm pit, and arms
- [ ] Loss of the lateral (outer) one-third of the eyebrows
- [ ] Loss or thinning of eyelashes
- [ ] Low blood pressure
- [ ] Low body temperature

- [ ] Mild elevation of liver enzymes, which affects liver function
- [ ] Morning stiffness
- [ ] Muscle and joint pain
- [ ] Muscle cramps
- [ ] Muscle weakness
- [ ] Muscular pain
- [ ] Nocturia (urinary frequency during the night)
- [ ] Nutritional imbalances
- [ ] Painful menstrual cycles
- [ ] Parathesias (numbness and tingling of the extremities)
- [ ] PMS
- [ ] Poor circulation
- [ ] Poor night vision
- [ ] Produces abnormal waves on EEG
- [ ] Puffy face
- [ ] Recurrent miscarriages
- [ ] Reduced heart rate
- [ ] Rough, dry skin
- [ ] Sleep apnea
- [ ] Slow movements
- [ ] Slow speech
- [ ] Slower reflexes
- [ ] Swollen body, especially the legs, feet, hands, and abdomen
- [ ] Swollen eyelids
- [ ] Tinnitus (ringing in ears)
- [ ] Vitamin $B_{12}$ deficiency
- [ ] Weight gain
- [ ] Yellowish coloring of the skin

# Thyroid Hormone and Iodine

Iodine, a chemical element, is particularly important when considering thyroid function. Iodine is an antibacterial, anticancer, antiparasitic, antiviral, and mucolytic agent.

Iodine is needed to maintain healthy breast tissue and nerve function, and it protects against toxic effects from radioactive material. According to the World Health Organization, up to 72 percent of the world's population is affected by an iodine deficiency disorder.

## ■ Causes of Iodine Deficiency

- Diets high in pasta and breads (which contain bromide)*
- Diets without ocean fish or sea vegetables (such as seaweed)
- Flouride use, which inhibits iodine binding
- Foods that interfere with iodine:
  Cabbage
  Cauliflower
  Rutabaga
  Soybeans
- Ground that is deplete in iodine

- Inadequate use of iodized salt (sea salt is not rich in iodine)
- Some medications:
  *Atrovent* inhaler (contains bromide)
  *FLONASE* (contains fluoride)
  *Flovent* (contains fluoride)
  *Ipratropium* nasal spray (contains bromide)
  *Pro-Banthine* (contains bromide)
- Splenda, a sugar substitute, which contains chlorinated table sugar
- Vegan and vegetarian diets

*Bromide binds to the iodine receptors and displaces the iodine.

Low thyroid levels can lead to other ailments and problems. For example, low thyroid hormone levels directly affect pregnenolone levels in hypothyroid patients (see section on pregnenolone, page 38). Mild thyroid dysfunction is also associated with heart disease.

Additionally, thyroid hormones also affect muscle metabolism. If your thyroid is not functioning optimally, you won't build muscle. As you are likely aware, your muscles are a major part of your body. Some muscles, like the heart, work within the body to pump blood, keeping the body functioning. Other muscles, like the bicep and triceps (in your arms) or the quadriceps (in your leg) serve locomotive purposes, causing movement.

Contrary to the foods that interfere with iodine, there are plenty of foods that are useful sources of iodine.

## ■ Food Sources of Iodine

- Beef
- Beef liver
- Bread, whole wheat
- Butter
- Cheese, cheddar
- Cheese, cottage
- Clams
- Cream

- Eggs
- Green peppers
- Haddock
- Halibut
- Lamb
- Lettuce
- Milk
- Oysters
- Peanuts

- Pineapple
- Pork
- Raisins
- Salmon
- Sardines (canned)
- Shrimp
- Spinach
- Tuna (canned)

Be aware, however, that if you intake too much iodine you can get acne. Too much iodine can also cause thyroiditis, an inflammation of the thyroid gland that results in overproduction of the thyroid hormone. Your healthcare practitioner can measure your iodine levels with a urine test.

If you need iodine replacement, it will most likely contain iodine and iodide. Iodine replacement comes in both a liquid and tablet form. Lugol's solution is a liquid iodine replacement. Iodoral is a tablet that replaces both iodine and iodide. About one-third of people treated for low thyroid function will need to have a lower dose of thyroid medication when the iodine deficiency is corrected.

## ■ Diseases and Conditions Associated With Hypothyroidism

- ADHD
- Ankylosing spondylitis, a disease where the spine becomes fused and the sufferer has a hard time moving
- Chronic fatigue/fibromyalgia
- Congestive heart failure

- Depression
- Elevated cholesterol
- Heart disease
- High C-reactive protein
- Increased homocysteine levels
- Insulin resistance

# Reverse T3

Reverse T3 is a measurement of inactive thyroid function. Reverse T3 has only 1 percent of the activity T3 does. It is an antagonist of T3, which means that the higher your reverse T3 level is, the lower your T3 level will be. T3 and reverse T3 bind to the same receptor sites, so they cannot both occupy these sites at the same time. This situation occurs due to a malfunction of the metabolism of T4. When your reverse T3 is high this is a medical syndrome now called "reverse T3 dominance."

The most common reason that reverse T3 levels become elevated is stress. When you are stressed, your cortisol levels rise. If you stay stressed all the time your cortiosl levels will stay elevated (see page 35). This phenomenon can cause your body to produce more reverse T3.

## ■ Causes of Reverse T3 Dominance

- Autoimmune disease
- Exposure to electromagnetic radiation
- Exposure to environmental toxins such as chemical pollutants, pesticides, mercury, or fluoride
- Food deprivation
- High levels of stress
- Hormonal imbalances (such as high estrogen levels)
- Infections
- Nutritional deficiencies
- Poor liver function

When you have a high reverse T3 level, you can have any or all of the symptoms of hypothyroidism (low thyroid function) that have been discussed in this section. The most common symptom that I see in my

Decreased production of T3 can cause high cholesterol, because low levels of T3 cause less cholesterol to be removed from your blood. This causes an increase in bad cholesterol. People who have low thyroid levels have cholesterol levels that are 10 to 50 percent higher than people with normal thyroid function.

Inadequate thyroid function can stimulate CYP3A4, a part of the P450 system in the liver, which can cause an increase in production of 16-hydroxy estrone. It can also lead to a decrease in SHBG, which increases the bioavailable amount of E2 and testosterone in the body.

practice in patients who have high reverse T3 levels is weight gain. It is very difficult to lose weight and keep it off if your reverse T3 levels remain elevated. Unfortunately, weight gain is also very discouraging. It may make dealing with other problems seem more difficult.

Additionally, when your reverse T3 level is high your body temperature goes down. This slows the action of many enzymes in your body, which can lead to a syndrome called "multiple enzyme dysfunction."

### ■ Symptoms of Multiple Enzyme Dysfunction

| □ Anxiety | □ Headache | □ Panic attacks |
| □ Fatigue | □ Irritability | □ PMS |
| □ Fluid retention | □ Migraine headaches | |

Consequently, it is very important to have your reverse T3 levels measured. Some scientists believe that the best indicator of thyroid function is the ratio between T3 and reverse T3 since this ratio measures the tissue levels of thyroid hormone.

High levels of reverse T3 can be treated nutritionally. Taking the nutrients that aid the conversion of T4 to T3 (see page 51) is very helpful. Selenium, zinc, vitamins $B_6$ and $B_{12}$, iron (if levels are low), vitamin D, and iodine have all been found to be helpful. If you are taking T4 supplementation, discontinuing it can also increase T3 and lower reverse T3 levels. However, do not do this without the aid of a physician. Taking a T3 prescription will also increase T3 levels and decrease reverse T3. Furthermore, if you have elevated cortisol levels, lowering them to normal will also diminish your reverse T3.

Decreased thyroid levels can be caused by a variety of factors. Sometimes, a deficiency of certain minerals can lead to low thyroid production. There are many elements that can have similar consequences when they are not at their proper levels.

### ■ Nutritional Deficiencies That Can Cause a Decrease in T4 Production

| • Copper | • Vitamins A, $B_2$, $B_3$, $B_6$, and C | • Zinc |

## T4 to T3 Conversion

Your body also needs to be able to convert T4 to T3. T3 is the more active form of thyroid hormone. This conversion requires an enzyme called 5'diodinase.

The inability to convert T4 to T3 will lead to symptoms of thyroid hormone loss. As discussed earlier, T4 also sometimes converts into reverse T3, which can also lead to symptoms of thyroid loss.

### ■ Effects of Decreased T3 (or Increased Reverse T3)

- Aging
- Chronic fatigue
- Diabetes
- Fasting
- Fibromyalgia
- IL-6, TNF-alpha, IFN-2 (immune system factors)
- Increased catecholamines (epinephrine and norepinephrine)
- Increased free radicals
- Infections
- Prolonged illness
- Stress
- Toxic metal exposure
- Yo-yo dieting

As mentioned, the conversion of T4 to T3 cannot take place without 5'diodinase, an enzyme. There are many factors that can affect your body's production of this enzyme.

### ■ Factors That Affect 5'diodinase Production

- Cadmium, mercury, or lead toxicity
- Chronic illness
- Decreased kidney or liver function
- Elevated cortisol
- Estrogen excess
- Herbicides, pesticides
- High carbohydrate diet
- Inadequate protein intake
- Oral contraceptives
- Polycyclic aromatic hydrocarbons
- Selenium deficiency
- Starvation
- Stress

There are other factors besides insufficient 5'diodinase levels that can lead to an inability to convert T4 to T3.

## ■ Additional Factors That Cause an Inability to Convert T4 to T3

- Aging
- Alpha-lipotic acid (too much)
- Calcium excess
- Certain medications:
  - Beta-blockers
  - Birth control pills
  - Chemotherapy
  - Estrogen
  - Lithium
  - Phenytoin
  - Theophylline
- Copper excess
- Deficiency in the following nutrients:
  - Iodine
  - Iron
  - Selenium
  - Vitamins A, $B_2$, $B_6$, and $B_{12}$
  - Zinc
- Diabetes

- Dietary factors:
  - Cruciferous vegetables (too many)
  - Excessive alcohol intake
  - Low carbohydrate diet
  - Low fat diet
  - Low protein diet
  - Soy
  - Walnuts
- Dioxins
- Fluoride
- Inadequate production of adrenal hormones (DHEA, cortisol)
- Lead
- Mercury
- PCBs
- Pesticides
- Phtalates (chemicals added to plastics)
- Radiation
- Stress
- Surgery

Iron deficiency and physical inactivity impair your body's response to T3. These factors will also cause you to have symptoms of low thyroid.

On the contrary, there are factors that will increase the conversion of T4 to T3 if there is not enough T3 being made by your body.

## ■ Factors That Increase the Conversion of T4 to T3*

- Ashwaganda
- Glucagon
- Growth hormone

- High protein diet
- Insulin
- Iodine

*You may notice that some of the same things that decrease the conversion of T4 to T3 also increase it. This is due to the fact that it is important to have the right amount of these nutrients, herbs, and hormones in your body. Too much or too little will affect thyroid production and, subsequently, function.*

- Iron
- Melatonin
- Potassium
- Selenium

- Testosterone
- Tyrosine
- Vitamins A, B$_2$, and E
- Zinc

## Hypothyroidism Fixes

When your doctor sends you for thyroid studies, your entire thyroid panel should be measured—this includes your free T3, reverse T3, free T4, TSH, and your thyroid antibodies. (Tests for T1 and T2 are still in experimental stages and are not available.) If your antibodies are too high, they can stop the thyroid hormone from attaching to the thyroid receptors. Consequently, you can get symptoms of decreased thyroid function—even when your blood levels are adequate. Thyroid antibodies can be elevated due to trauma, poor function of your gut, inflammation, and thyroid degeneration.

Thyroid antibodies are measured by blood. They include thyroid peroxidase antibody (TPOab), thyroglobulin antibody (Tgab), and thyroid stimulating hormone receptor antibody (TRab). If your antibodies are elevated and you have hypothyroidism, this is called "Hashimoto's thyroiditis," which is an autoimmune disease. Autoimmune diseases occur when the body is trying to attack itself. With Hashimoto's thyroiditis, the body is literally attacking the thyroid gland and your body is not producing enough thyroid hormone due to this attack.

There are a number of different hypothyroidism treatments out there. *Synthroid* and Levothyroxine are both comprised of only T4. *Armour Thyroid* is made up of T3, T4, T1, T2, and other substances that help the body convert T4 into T3, such as calcitonin, selenium, and diuretic effect. Some physicians feel that *Armour Thyroid* is not consistent from dose-to-dose. However, there has never been a complaint to the FDA concerning the inconsistency of *Armour Thyroid*.

If you are diagnosed with hypothyroidism, it is important that your doctor replace both T4 and T3. If you only have your T4 pathway replaced, you may still experience low thyroid symptoms. Replacing T3 and T4 has been found to be more effective than replacing T4 alone in most people. One study revealed that 35 percent of people on T4 and T3 replacement scored better on mental agility tests than people who were just taking T4. Of these people, 67 percent stated they had an improvement in mood and physical health. Likewise, benefits have been shown by adding T3 for patients already on T4, with the patients reporting better moods and brain function.

You can replace both thyroid pathways by adding T3 (Cytomel) to T4 (*Synthroid*, etc.). *Armour Thyroid*, which is four parts T4 to one part T3, may not be the right ratio for everyone. If this is the case, your healthcare practitioner can have the T3 and T4 compounded so that your dose is literally made for you, the same way your natural hormones are customized for your needs.

Thyroid medication should be taken on an empty stomach. Eat no food or vitamins for one hour prior to or after taking the medication, since calcium (which is in many foods) interferes with the absorption of thyroid replacement. It is not just dairy foods that are a problem—many other foods contain calcium. Additional things that alter thyroid absorption are ferrous sulfate (iron), aluminum hydroxide-containing antacids, and medications such as sucrafate and bile acid sequestrants.

You may have a hard time tolerating thyroid replacement if you have adrenal fatigue. This is why you should always have your adrenal health evaluated before you are prescribed thyroid medication. Adrenal dysfunction should be treated before you start thyroid replacement. (For more on adrenal fatigue, see page 32.) For this reason, it is important you see a healthcare practitioner who has completed a two-year fellowship in Metabolic/Anti-Aging Medicine and has a Master's Degree in Metabolic and Nutritional Medicine. (For information on how to locate a fellowship-trained/Master's Degree healthcare professional, see the Resources section on page 183.)

Some people develop thyroid resistance due to excess adrenalin production. This is where thyroid receptors (particularly receptors for T3) become desensitized and do not work as well. So, your levels of T3 may be normal or even high, but because the T3 is resistant, you may still have symptoms of low thyroid function. What may also occur is that you take thyroid medication but your body doesn't tolerate it. In this case, you will experience symptoms of too much thyroid hormone, such as a racing heart and headache. (For more on thyroid hormone excess, see page 54.) This is why it's important your healthcare practitioner always checks your adrenals before starting you on any thyroid treatment.

Additionally, low magnesium levels may also interfere with your ability to tolerate thyroid replacement. Chronic exposure to mold can have similar effects. Also, if your gut is healthy, it is easier for your body to assimilate the medication. How you respond to hormone replacement is also associated with your own unique genetic makeup. Therefore, if you are sensitive to thyroid hormone replacement, you may have a genetic problem with detoxifying (which is discussed on page 12).

Zinc supplementation has been shown to help with thyroid metabolism. Likewise, taking selenium has been shown in a clinical study to help normalize thyroid function.

You may find that you are experiencing symptoms of hypothyroidism, but your blood levels of thyroid hormone are normal. In this case, you should check your basal body temperature, which is the lowest temperature your body reaches during rest. If your basal body temperature is low (below 97.4°F), then you may benefit from a low dose of Armour thyroid, even though your blood level is within a "normal range," but not an optimal range.

To check your basal body temperature, take your temperature under your arm for ten minutes when you wake up in the morning before you get out of bed. Record your temperature for three days. If you are menstruating, check your basal body temperature during your cycle. Ovulation can change your basal body temperature. The body's temperature goes up with ovulation so that is why it is not recommended to measure basal body temperature during that time. There may be an elevation in temperature due to ovulation, which can skew results if a person really has low temperature, which can indicate low thyroid function.

## HYPERTHYROIDISM (EXCESSIVE THYROID FUNCTION)

Contrary to hypothyroidism, your body can produce too much thyroid hormone. This is called hyperthyroidism. The most common cause of hyperthyroidism is Grave's disease (also known as toxic diffuse goiter). Grave's disease is an autoimmune disease where the body is trying to attack the thyroid gland. This is very much like Hashimoto's thyroiditis, although with Grave's disease the amount of thyroid hormone is being overproduced due to destruction by the autoimmune process.

Grave's disease is more common in women than in men. It can occur at any age but is frequently diagnosed between the ages of thirty and forty.

There are other less common causes of overproduction of thyroid hormones. Taking too much thyroid medication is one of these, and is called factitious thyroiditis. If you have a pituitary or thyroid tumor, your body may make an excess of thyroid hormones. You may also have a nodule on your thyroid that overproduces thyroid hormone. This is called "toxic nodular goiter." Lastly, some medications can cause drug interactions that can result in an abundance of thyroid production. If you are taking levothyroxine (T4) and the medication Indinavir, this can occur.

## ■ Symptoms of Hyperthyroidism

- ☐ Chest pain
- ☐ Excessive sweating
- ☐ Fatigue at the end of the day
- ☐ Hair loss
- ☐ Heart racing
- ☐ Heat intolerance (feeling warm all the time)
- ☐ Heightened anxiety, irritability, moodiness, or depression
- ☐ Increased bowel movements

- ☐ Insomnia
- ☐ Light or absent menstrual cycles
- ☐ Muscle weakness
- ☐ Puffiness around the eyes
- ☐ Shortness of breath
- ☐ Staring gaze
- ☐ Thickening of the skin of the lower leg
- ☐ Warm, moist skin
- ☐ Weight loss

If you have hyperthyroidism, an endocrinologist can use many treatment modalities. If you have mild hyperthyroidism, the amino acid carnitine at 3,000 to 4,000 mg a day may be an effective treatment.

There are also foods that suppress the production of thyroid hormone.

## ■ Foods That Suppress Thyroid Hormone Production

- • Cruciferous vegetables, such as:
  Broccoli
  Brussels sprouts
  Cabbage
  Cauliflower
  Kale
- • Leafy green vegetables
- • Peaches
- • Pears
- • Soybeans

Hyperthyroidism can be a life-threatening disease, so it should always be managed by your doctor. If your thyroid hormone production is more than slightly elevated, your healthcare practitioner may need to prescribe a medication.

### ■ Medications Used to Treat Hyperthyroidism

- Beta blockers
- Dexamethasone
- Esmolol
- Guanethidine
- Methimazole
- Potassium iodide
- Propylthiouracil
- Radioactive iodine

If you have mild hyperthyroidism, a high dose of carnitine (an amino acid) of 3,000 to 4,000 mg a day may be helpful. Some people require surgery to treat their hyperthyroidism. However, most people with hyperthyroidism are treated with radioactive iodine, which is given as a capsule. Within six weeks to six months, thyroid function is ablated. This commonly leads to hypothyroidism, or low thyroid function, which will require thyroid medication.

## OTHER TESTS OF THYROID FUNCTION

Besides blood studies, your doctor can do some other tests to look at thyroid function.

- Thyroid scans. Thyroid scans are common tests that are done to determine if you have a thyroid nodule (a lump that arises on the thyroid gland) and if the nodule is hot or cold. If you have a goiter (enlargement of the thyroid gland) its size can be measured by a thyroid scan. If you have had thyroid cancer, then a thyroid scan can be used after surgery to see if you have a reoccurrence of cancer. Thyroid scans are also used to see if you have thyroid tissue located outside of the neck. The scan is done by giving a radioisotope (like radioactive iodine) and letting the thyroid gland (or thyroid tissue outside of the thyroid) take up the isotope.

- Thyroid ultrasounds. Thyroid ultrasounds are another method of testing thyroid function and assessing thyroid nodules. With this study, sound waves are used to tell if a thyroid nodule is solid or a cyst. However, this test will not tell your doctor if the nodule is cancerous or benign (non-cancerous). If your healthcare practitioner needs more information, you may be sent for a biopsy of your thyroid gland.

# MELATONIN

Melatonin is another hormone your body makes. It is made in the pineal gland in the brain, the retina of the eye, the gastrointestinal tract, and the white blood cells. Melatonin sets your body's twenty-four-hour cycle. What this means is that adequate levels of melatonin keep your body running on a day-to-day basis. Melatonin causes drowsiness and lowers your body temperature when it's time for you to sleep, and it also helps you wake up by resetting your daily biological time clock.

Melatonin is made from the amino acid tryptophan, which is also used to make serotonin. Therefore, when melotonin levels go up, serotonin levels go down. If you eat too many high-sugar carbohydrates, you will make less melatonin because carbohydrates shift your amino acid balance to make more serotonin.

Your body needs B vitamins in order to convert tryptophan into melatonin. Therefore, if you do not have an adequate intake of vitamin B-rich foods or you do not take a supplement, your body may be deficient in melatonin.

Melatonin serves more purposes than simply monitoring your internal clock. It has an influence on many of your body's functions.

### ■ Influences of Melatonin in Your Body

- Affects the release of sex hormones
- Aids the immune system in working normally in the body
- Antioxidant activity (it is more potent than Vitamin C or E)
- Blocks estrogen from binding to estrogen receptors
- Decreases cortisol levels
- Helps balance the stress response
- Helps prevent cancer
- Improves mood
- Improves sleep quality
- Increases the action of benzodiazepine medications
- Stimulates the parathyroid gland, which regulates bone formation
- Stimulates the production of growth hormone

Recent studies are suggesting that melatonin and testosterone regulate the synthesis of each other. There are also some studies that show that if you do not sleep at least seven hours a day you increase your risk of several diseases, including heart disease. In fact, additional studies have revealed that melatonin levels are lower in patients with heart disease than in healthy people. The hormones in the body really are a symphony. If your melatonin level is low and your quality of sleep is poor, this directly affects the amount of growth hormone that your body makes.

Growth hormone is one of the hormones in the body that helps you look and feel younger. So, if you are not sleeping for an adequate amount of time and you are not getting enough REM sleep (deep sleep), your body literally ages.

Melatonin deficiencies can be caused by a variety of factors. A lot of medications can lead to deficiencies in melatonin.

## ■ Causes of Melatonin Deficiency

| | | |
|---|---|---|
| • Alcohol | Clonidine | Methylcobalamine |
| • Caffeine | Dexamethasone | Metoprolol |
| • Electromagnetic | Diazepam | Nicardipine |
|   fields | Diltiazem | Nifedipine |
| • Medications, such as: | Filodipine | Nimodipine |
|   Acetaminophen | Flunitrazepam | Nisoldipine |
|   Alcohol | Fluoxetine | Nitrendipine |
|   Aprazolam | Ibuprofen | Prazosin |
|   Aspirin | Indomethacin | Propanolol |
|   Atenolol | Interleukin-2 | Reserpine |
|   Benserazide | Isradapine | Ridazolol |
|   Bepridil | Luzindole | • Tobacco |

Naturally, like the other hormones, you can experience side effects if your melatonin levels are too high as well.

## ■ Symptoms of Excess Melatonin Production

☐ Daytime sleepiness/fatigue

☐ Depression

☐ Headaches

☐ Increase in cortisol, which can increase fat storage

☐ Intense dreaming/nightmares

☐ Suppression of serotonin, which will increase carbohydrate cravings

## ■ Causes of Excess Melatonin Production

- Exercise
- Foods, such as:
  - Bananas
  - Barley
  - Cherries
  - Ginger
  - Oats

- Rice
- Sweet corn
- Tomatoes
- Walnuts
- Medications, such as:
  - *Clorgyline*
  - *Desipramine*

- *Fluvoxamine*
- *Thorazine*
- *Tranylcypromine*
- St. John's wort
- Taking melatonin as a supplement

If you take melatonin and your levels become too high, you may suppress estrogen and testosterone in your body. In contrast, if you have too little melatonin you may increase the risk of age-related diseases (as discussed earlier in this section). Consequently, it is very important to have the right amount of this hormone in your body.

Melatonin is an immune stimulator. Therefore, if you have an autoimmune disease you should not take melatonin, unless instructed to do so by your doctor. Autoimmune diseases cause your body to be in a state where your immune system is overactive. Taking too much melatonin may make the autoimmune disease worse. Furthermore, you should not take melatonin if you are pregnant, breastfeeding, on prescription steroids, are depressed, have a mental illness, have lymphoma, or suffer from leukemia.

At menopause, there is a decline in melatonin secretion. Therefore, you should have your melatonin levels measured if you have insomnia, if you have cancer, or if you are perimenopausal or menopausal.

# PROLACTIN

Prolactin is a hormone your body produces. It is made by your pituitary gland, which is located in your brain. Prolactin regulates nursing after childbirth. It also decreases ovarian hormone production after delivery, which helps prevent a new pregnancy while you are still nursing your baby.

When prolactin levels drop too low, you are unable to nurse due to decreased milk production.

## ■ Causes of Prolactin Deficiency

- Head injury
- Infection (such as tuberculosis)
- Infiltrative diseases
- Parasellar diseases (such as a brain tumor)
- Pituitary tumor (or treatment of tumor)
- Sheehan's syndrome (a condition affecting women who experience life-threatening blood loss during or after childbirth)

## ■ Symptoms of Excess Prolactin

- ☐ Bone loss
- ☐ Breast enlargement
- ☐ Depression
- ☐ Headaches
- ☐ Infertility
- ☐ Milky discharge from the breast
- ☐ Menstrual irregularity
- ☐ Muscle loss
- ☐ Suppressed ovarian function with a decrease in ovarian hormone production
- ☐ Weight gain

## ■ Causes of Excess Prolactin

- Excessive exercise
- Hypothyroidism
- Menopause
- Pituitary tumor
- Some medications, such as:
  Anticonvulsants (*Depakote*)
  Antinausea medications (*Compazine, Reglan*)
  H2 blockers (*Pepcid, Tagamet*)
  Neuroleptic medications (*Haldol, Mellaril, Risperdal, Seroquel,* and others)
  SSRI anti-depressants (*Celexa, Luvox, Paxil, Prozac, Zoloft*)
  Tricyclic anti-depressants
- Stress

# Ailments and Problems

# Introduction to Part II

For many years, science has ignored the role that hormonal function plays in the relationship between a woman and her body. Issues such as insomnia or anxiety may be related to hormonal levels. How well you maintain vision, memory, and mobility are also related to optimal hormonal function. Even your risk of heart disease and stroke can be related, in part, to your hormonal levels.

Recent research has brought about many new medications and treatments to decrease your risk factors for disease and to help you live a healthier and longer life. An example of this is Metabolic/Anti-Aging Medicine. Metabolic/Anti-Aging Medicine is not a complementary or alternative specialty. It is a specialty that looks at the metabolism of the body and how the body works. It takes into consideration that medical problems are highly individualized. The same symptoms in two different people may mean entirely different things.

Part II of this book takes a glimpse at the ailments and problems that can occur if your hormones are not all balanced. Many common problems that women experience—such as PMS, premenstrual dysphoric disorder (PMDD), postpartum depression, endometriosis, bladder problems, migraine headaches, and vulvodynia—will be discussed in this section.

One size does *not* fit all when it comes to your medical treatment. As always, working with a healthcare professional is suggested. Additionally, when taking supplements, always consume them with a full glass of water.

It is also important you note the following precautions, along with the considerations given for each supplement. The dosages listed are intended for adults without kidney or liver disease. If you have kidney or liver disease, you may need to take lower dosages of most supplements, and should consult your doctor before embarking on any nutritional program. Similarly, if you are pregnant or nursing, consult your doctor before following any of these protocols. If you are taking *Coumadin* or any other blood thinner, your dosage of certain nutrients must be lower than what is suggested. Please ask your physician for help determining the appropriate dosage. If you are having surgery, do not take any nutrients (except for the surgery pre- and post-operative protocol that your doctor gives you) for two weeks before and one week after your surgery date.

## ACIDITY

*See* Osteoporosis.

## ACNE

*See* Cystic Acne; Polycystic Ovarian Syndrome (PCOS); Premenstrual Syndrome (PMS); Skin Problems.

## ADENOCARCINOMA

*See* Diethylstilbestrol (DES) Babies.

## AGE SPOTS

*See* Skin Problems.

## ALLERGIES

*See* Skin Problems.

## ANXIETY

*See* Premenstrual Dysphoric Disorder (PMDD); Premenstrual Syndrome (PMS).

## ARTERIOSCLEROSIS

*See* Heart Disease.

## BACK PAIN

*See* Endometriosis; Osteoporosis; Premenstrual Syndrome (PMS).

## BLADDER PROBLEMS

Like the vagina, the bladder has estrogen receptors. When your estrogen levels start to decline, you may have urinary leakage (incontinence). Sometimes, a loss of muscle tone will occur, which means you will not be able to hold your urine. Also as a result of this, your bladder may become more sensitive to the stimuli that urge you to urinate. Estrogen replacement therapy may significantly help bladder symptoms.

Drinking caffeine for some people can also cause urgency (the sensation that you have to urinate immediately) or incontinence. Dyes that contain tartrazine (such as FD&C yellow #5) in foods, drinks, and even medications or vitamins can irritate the bladder.

## BLOATING

*See* Menopause; Premenstrual Dysphoric Disorder (PMDD); Premenstrual Syndrome (PMS).

## BLOOD CLOTS

*See* Heart Disease.

## BONE FRACTURES

*See* Osteoporosis.

## BREAST CANCER

*See* Cancer.

## BREAST SWELLING/TENDERNESS

*See* Fibrocystic Breast Disease; Menopause; Premenstrual Dysphoric Disorder (PMDD); Premenstrual Syndrome (PMS).

# C-REACTIVE PROTEIN (CRP) TOXICITY

*See* Heart Disease.

# CALCIUM DEFICIENCY

*See* Osteoporosis.

# CANCER

This section is not designed to be an extensive, exhaustive look at the prevention of every type of cancer. However, without including a section on the most common types of cancer women experience, the text seemed incomplete.

This section will focus on breast, ovarian, uterine, and cervical cancers.

Additionally, this chapter will focus on preventing cancer, rather than treating the disease.

## ■ Preventing Cancer

Because many elements of daily life serve as risk factors for cancer, it should come as no surprise that studies have shown most cancers are preventable by making lifestyle changes.

Exercising has been shown to decrease the risk of all cancers by almost 50 percent. Furthermore, exercise can help with some other risk factors for cancer, such as poor diet, being overweight, and smoking.

Vitamin D affects at least 200 genes. Some of these genes regulate cancer cell growth and differentiation. They also regulate cancer cell death and limit the growth of tumor blood supplies (angiogenesis).

| SUPPLEMENTATION TO PREVENT CANCER | | |
| --- | --- | --- |
| Supplements | Dosage | Considerations |
| Vitamin D | About 1,000 international units (IU) a day, but the dosage is best determined by a lab measurement | Can reduce the risk of developing cancer by 60 to 77 percent |

# Risk Factors for Cancer

There are many elements of daily life that can serve as risk factors for various types of cancer.

According to numerous medical studies, following a high glycemic index diet can increase the risk of many types of cancer, including breast, endometrial, stomach, and colorectal. The glycemic index ranks carbohydrates in the diet according to their effect on blood sugar levels. Make sure you always eat a low glycemic index program.

Furthermore, being overweight increases your risk of many kinds of cancers. One study, which followed over 900,000 women and men over a sixteen-year period, showed that the heavier participants were, the higher their death rate for all forms of cancer was. Overweight women had a 62 percent higher death rate than those with "normal" weights, and overweight men had a 52 percent higher death rate. Being overweight can also increase your levels of estrogen and insulin, which may increase the rate of cancer cell growth. Endometrial and gallbladder cancer risks are five times greater if you are overweight.

Nutritional deficiencies of some vitamins have been associated with an increased risk of several types of cancers. For example, if you have a higher vitamin D level you have a markedly reduced risk of developing cancer of the breast, uterus, ovary, cervix, colon, esophagus, pancreas, rectum, bladder, kidney, or lung. You also have a reduced risk of developing non-Hodgkin's lymphoma and multiple myeloma. Consequently, a deficiency in vitamin D increases your risk of developing the types of cancer mentioned. However, medical studies have shown that your vitamin D level must be optimal and not just normal in order to reap this nutrient's benefits. An optimal level of vitamin D is 55 nanograms per milliliter (ng/mL) or greater.

## BREAST CANCER

Breast cancer is the second leading cause of cancer death in women (lung cancer is the first) and accounts for about 30 percent of all newly diagnosed cancers in U.S. women. There are many risk factors that have been shown to increase your risk of developing breast cancer.

Additionally, clinical trials have shown that diet may contribute to between 30 and 50 percent of breast cancer occurrences. Studies have

If all people had vitamin D levels of 55 ng/mL, it is projected that in North America alone, 85,000 cases of breast cancer and 60,000 cases of colon cancer would be prevented annually.

Some researchers believe cancer may be linked to a dysfunction of the mitochondria, which are the "engines" of your cells. Many cancer patients have low levels of coenzyme Q-10, one of the main nutrients that fuels the mitochondria. Raising Q-10 levels in cancer patients has been associated with an increase in survival rate. Therefore, you want to make sure that your body has enough coenzyme Q-10.

Coenzyme Q-10 levels decrease with true exercise, aging, and some medications. True exercise is doubling your pulse for twenty minutes. Exercising is great for you, but your body needs fuel in order to exercise, and coenzyme Q-10 is one of the fueling sources used. The body requires tyrosine, phenylalanine, vitamins C, $B_2$, $B_3$, $B_5$, $B_6$, $B_{12}$, and folate to make coenzyme Q-10. Consequently, a deficiency in any of these nutrients may lead to low coenzyme Q-10 levels in your body.

Prolonged stress has been shown to be a risk factor for many cancers. The people who are most likely to suffer stress are those who avoid conflict, are overly nice, and use denial as a coping mechanism. These types of people tend to suppress their emotions, especially anger.

High levels of certain enzymes can also increase your risk of developing cancer. Some cancers—such as endometrial, cervical, breast, ovarian, colon, lung, and glioma—are associated with high levels of COX and LOX, enzymes that are part of the inflammatory pathway. Nutrients such as ginkgo, curcumin, kaempferol, and quercetin increase your levels of COX and LOX.

Women who took DES (see page 78) have a higher risk of developing cancer. Additionally, other studies have shown that daughters of women who took DES have an increased risk of cervical, breast, and vaginal cancers.

shown that eating a low glycemic index diet is more protective against breast cancer than eating high glycemic index meals. If you eat a high glycemic diet *and* a diet that is too high in red meat, you may increase your risk of developing breast cancer by as much as 60 percent, according to one medical trial. If you factor out the hormonally-related breast cancers, the people in this trial that ate a standard American diet (high glycemic and high in red meat) had a 90 percent increase in developing breast cancer.

---

# Risk Factors for Breast Cancer

- Alcohol consumption
- Cigarette smoking
- Diet
- Estrogen dominance

- Exposure to DES (see page 78 for more information)
- Lack of exercise
- Night-shift work

---

Even more compelling is that over 90 percent of breast tumors are insulin-receptor positive. This means that the amount of sugary or high glycemic index foods that you eat is directly related to the development and progression of breast cancer.

For some people, alcohol intake is a risk factor for breast cancer. Moderate intake of alcohol (one glass of wine, one beer, or one ounce of alcohol per day) does not seem to increase your risk of developing breast cancer. Drinking more than this amount, however, increases your risk. A trial conducted on premenopausal women required the women to consume two drinks a day for three menstrual cycles and then no alcohol at all for another three cycles. The results showed that the intake of alcohol was associated with an increase in total estrogen levels and the amount of bioavailable estrogens. In other words, alcohol intake may enhance mammary gland susceptibility to cancer, increase mammary carcinogen DNA damage, and create greater metastatic potential of the breast cancer cells.

Cigarette smoking has been associated with an increased risk in breast cancer. If you smoke, this is yet another reason you should quit.

Several medical studies have shown that women who work the graveyard shift for an extended period of time have an increased risk of developing breast cancer. One trial revealed a 60 percent increase. You may want to take 1 to 3 mg of melatonin when you go to bed if you do night-shift work (regardless of when you are going to bed) to offset the increased risk in breast cancer.

## ■ Preventing Breast Cancer

There are things you can do to prevent or decrease your risk of developing this disease. Studies have shown that eating cruciferous vegetables (broccoli, cauliflower, Brussels sprouts, cabbage, and kale) decreases your risk of developing breast cancer, since their consumption improves the breakdown of estrogen in your body into components that decrease your risk of breast cancer.

A Mediterranean diet (a diet high in omega-3 fatty acids and vegetables) has been associated with a decrease risk in many diseases, including breast cancer. One study found that women who consume olive oil have a 25 percent lower risk of developing breast cancer. The intake of dietary lignans found in flax seed have also been known to decrease breast cancer risk.

As stated earlier, optimal levels of vitamin D in your body decrease your risk of developing breast cancer. Studies have shown that a lower intake of vitamin D and calcium can result in denser tissue (as revealed by mammography). This can also increase your risk of developing breast cancer.

Studies have shown that vigorous exercise decreases your risk of developing breast cancer by 30 percent.

Taking EPA/DHA (fish oil) may help prevent cancer, according to a clinical trial comparing women with invasive breast cancer and women with benign breast conditions. Women in this trial who had invasive breast cancer had much lower levels of DHA than women without breast cancer.

As stated earlier, prolonged stress is a risk factor for many cancers—but this is especially true of breast cancer. Stress that occurs for a long time reduces methylation of estrogens so that they are not broken down in the body into the "good" estrogens. This occurs because the methyl groups that are involved in methylation get used up by the body to make adrenaline when you are stressed. Some foods have been found to be helpful in improving methylation. Green leafy vegetables, legumes, citrus, berries, and nuts would be good choices for this.

| SUPPLEMENTATION TO PREVENT BREAST CANCER | |
|---|---|
| Supplements | Dosage |
| Calcium | 800 to 1,200 mg a day |
| EPA/DHA (fish oil) | 2,000 mg a day |
| Sulforaphane | 20 to 30 mg a day |
| Vitamin D | Dosage is best determined by a lab measurement |

## CERVICAL CANCER

Cervical cancer is the fifth leading cause of cancer deaths in women overall. But, it is the second most common cancer women between the ages of fifteen and thirty-four suffer from. Since the development of the Papani-

## Risk Factors for Cervical Cancer

The biggest risk factor to the development of cervical cancer is to be infected with the human papillomavirus (HPV, see page 75). There are several other major risk factors that have been elucidated that increase your risk of developing cervical cancer.

- Age
- Being a DES baby
- Birth control pill use
- Immunosuppression (compromised immune system)

- Nutritional deficiencies
- Sexual history
- Smoking

colaou (Pap) smear in the 1940s as an effective screening tool, the incidence of cervical cancer in the United States has decreased by 75 percent and the death rate continues to decline as well.

Women who have sexual intercourse before the age of eighteen, have multiple sexual partners, or who have had a child before the age of sixteen have a higher risk of developing cancer of the cervix.

Age plays a role in the development of cervical cancer along with how invasive the cancer may be. The risk of developing invasive cancer of the cervix increases after age twenty-five. Also, your odds of dying of cervical cancer increase as you age.

Birth control pills deplete the body of very important nutrients, such as vitamin $B_6$ and beta-carotene, vitamin C, folate, riboflavin, vitamin $B_{12}$, magnesium, selenium, and tyrosine. The use of birth control pills has been associated with an elevated risk of developing cervical dysplasia (precancerous lesion of the cervix). Clinical trials have shown that women who use birth control pills for more than five years may have an increased risk of cervical cancer. Some of the increased risk may be secondary to nutritional deficiencies caused by the use of birth control pills. Therefore, if you are taking birth control pills, make sure that you supplement with a pharmaceutical-grade multivitamin and/or a good B complex vitamin.

Smoking increases your risk of developing cervical cancer. In fact, women who smoke are twice as likely to develop cervical cancer than those who do not smoke.

Some nutritional deficiencies are linked to the development of cervical cancer. A clinical trial showed that women with low vitamin C intake were

10 times more likely to develop cervical cancer than women who ate foods that were higher in vitamin C. Other studies have shown that if you eat a diet low in vitamins $B_1$, $B_2$, and $B_{12}$, you may have an increased risk of developing cervical dysplasia. The same study also showed that women who were at high risk for developing cervical cancer or who were diagnosed with the disease had much lower levels of beta-carotene, lycopene, canthaxanthin, and alpha-tocopherol (a kind of vitamin E) than the control group.

## ■ Preventing Cervical Cancer

Abstinence or being in a monogamous relationship will dramatically decrease your risk of getting cervical cancer.

| SUPPLEMENTATION TO PREVENT CERVICAL CANCER | | |
|---|---|---|
| Supplements | Dosage | Considerations |
| B-vitamin complex | Dosage is best determined by a lab measurement | |
| Folate | 800 micrograms a day | Higher doses may be used under the direction of a physician—up to 3 mg a day |
| Vitamin C | 1,000 to 2,000 mg a day | |

## OVARIAN CANCER

Unfortunately, only about 20 percent of all cases of ovarian cancer are detected before the tumor growth has spread beyond the ovaries. A woman's chance of surviving ovarian cancer is better if the cancer is found early on.

## ■ Preventing Ovarian Cancer

Supplementation with certain nutrients may play a preventive role against ovarian cancer.

| SUPPLEMENTATION TO PREVENT OVARIAN CANCER | |
|---|---|
| Supplements | Dosage |
| Beta-cryptoxanthin | Dosage should be determined by a physician |
| Lutein | 6 to 12 mg |
| Lycopene | 10 mg |

# Risk Factors for Ovarian Cancer

- Age. Ovarian cancer is not common in women under the age of forty. Therefore, age is considered a risk factor for this type of cancer.

- Diet and nutrition also play a role in whether you have an increased risk of developing ovarian cancer. Studies have shown that women who consume dairy (quantities vary depending on the study) have a 44 percent greater risk of developing ovarian cancer.

- Inflammation. Studies have shown that elevated levels of COX-2 (an inflammatory marker) are present in people with ovarian cancer. Additionally, if one of your close family members had ovarian cancer, you are at a higher risk of developing it yourself.

## UTERINE CANCER

Uterine cancer is cancer of the uterus. It is the most common form of cancer of the female tract.

Endometrial cancer is a form of uterine cancer. It occurs in the lining of the uterus and is the most common form of cancer of the uterus. Uterine cancer usually occurs after menopause.

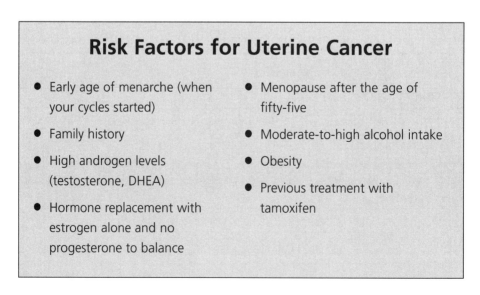

# Risk Factors for Uterine Cancer

- Early age of menarche (when your cycles started)

- Family history

- High androgen levels (testosterone, DHEA)

- Hormone replacement with estrogen alone and no progesterone to balance

- Menopause after the age of fifty-five

- Moderate-to-high alcohol intake

- Obesity

- Previous treatment with tamoxifen

### ■ Preventing Uterine Cancer

You can decrease your risk of uterine cancer by normalizing your weight and following a good diet. Also, exercise decreases your risk of developing this disease. Having normal melatonin levels or supplementing with melatonin when your levels are low also lowers your risk. Melatonin levels can be measured by a salivary test (see page 161 for details).

| SUPPLEMENTATION TO PREVENT UTERINE CANCER | | |
| --- | --- | --- |
| Supplements | Dosage | Considerations |
| Melatonin | Dosage should be measured by saliva testing | Too much melatonin can decrease the levels of serotonin in your body |

## CARCINOMA-IN-SITU

*See* Cervical Dysplasia (Abnormal Pap Smear).

## CARDIOVASCULAR DISEASE

*See* Heart Disease.

## CERVICAL CANCER

*See* Cancer; Cervical Dysplasia (Abnormal Pap Smear).

## CERVICAL DYSPLASIA (ABNORMAL PAP SMEAR)

Cervical dysplasia is the term used to describe abnormal cells on the surface of the cervix (the lowest part of the uterus). The changes in the cells are classified as mild, moderate, or severe. Mild dysplasia is called CIN I. Moderate to marked dysplasia is called CIN II. Finally, severe dysplasia to carcinoma-in-situ is called CIN III. (Carcinoma-in-situ is the term used to describe an early stage of a tumor, or cancer involving only the place in which it began.)

Cervical dysplasia doesn't cause health problems, but it is considered a pre-cancerous condition. It manifests prior to the development of cervi-

# Risk Factors for Cervical Dysplasia

There are several risk factors for cervical dysplasia. Numerous vitamin deficiencies have been associated with cervical dysplasia and cervical cancer. One study focusing on people with untreated cervical cancer revealed that at least 67 percent of the patients studied had at least one abnormal vitamin level. Of those patients, 38 percent had multiple vitamin deficiencies.

Nutrition plays a role in the risk factors for cervical cancer. Deficiencies of certain nutrients can increase your risk of developing cervical cancer, but proper levels of other nutrients can help decrease your risk. If your diet is rich in fruits, vegetables, and fiber, you will have a lower risk for this type of cancer.

## ■ Other Risk Factors for Cervical Cancer

- Having multiple sexual partners
- History of genital warts
- Infectious agents (chlamydia, herpes)
- Oral contraceptive use, long-term
- Pregnancy
- Sexual intercourse at an early age
- Sexually transmitted diseases (STDs), especially HIV infection and human papillomavirus
- Smoking

Deficiencies in certain nutrients can be risk factors for cervical dysplasia. For example, some studies show that women who have lower folic acid (folate) levels in their bodies have a higher rate of developing cervical dysplasia than women who have higher folate levels. Studies have also shown that folate depletion may correlate with abnormal growths in the cells of the cervix. Furthermore, research has also shown that supplementation of folate may reverse megaloblastic (large, dysfunctional red blood cells in people with disorders) changes in the tissue of the cervix. It's important to know that even if levels of folate in the blood appear to be adequate, levels of folate in the cervical tissue may be too low.

Cellular levels of beta-carotene (an organic compound and inactive form of vitamin A) are lower in women who have cervical dysplasia. An association has been found between the persistence of the HPV virus and lower concentrations of beta-carotene and other vitamin A derivatives, like beta-cryptoxanthin and lutein. Reduced levels of vitamin A (retinol) itself are also associated with an increased risk of developing cervical dysplasia. You should always consult a Metabolic/Anti-Aging physician for dosing (see the Resources section on page 183 for information on locating this doctor).

# HPV

If cervical dysplasia progresses into cervical cancer, most cases are associated with HPV, which is the most common STD. HPV is suggested to be the cause of 99.8 percent of the 320,000 cervical cancer cases that occur throughout the world each year.

There are more than 100 forms of HPV. Most of them have no harmful effects on the human body. Some can cause warts, but these types are low-risk. Some of the high-risk types of HPV cause cell changes that can eventually lead to cancer. Most types of HPV go away after eight to thirteen months, but other forms "hide," making it difficult to diagnose. At least 50 percent of sexually active men and women will contract some form of HPV in their lifetime. Some studies show that up to 80 percent of adults may be infected at some point in their life, with only 10 percent of those studied developing lesions on the cervix.

HPV can lead to many infections, including genital warts and cervical, vaginal, vulvar, or perianal dysplasia. These infections can progress into diseases or become cancerous. Some people have immune systems that protect against HPV developing into a disease process.

There are a few ways you can lower your risk of developing HPV. There is a vaccine available for women that protects against the four types of HPV that cause most cervical cancers. The vaccine is geared toward eleven and twelve-year-old girls, but is also recommended for any women between the ages of thirteen and twenty-six. The vaccine is associated with side effects in some people. Therefore, you should speak with your physician to see if the vaccine is right for you.

Using a condom during sexual intercourse also lowers the risk of developing HPV. Forgoing a condom not only increases your risk of developing HPV, it also increases your risk of developing cervical dysplasia, cervical cancer, and other STDs.

It is possible to catch HPV from examination tables, doorknobs, tanning beds, and other objects, but it is very hard to document. Having other infections such as chlamydia, herpes simplex, and bacterial vaginosis may also increase your risk of developing cervical dysplasia or cervical cancer.

Additionally, studies have shown that increased lycopene (a powerful antioxidant) levels in the body are associated with a resolution of HPV for some people. Lycopene isn't made in the body, but you can get it from many dietary sources, including tomatoes and tomato products, like soup, sauce, and ketchup.

cal cancer. Left untreated, cervical dysplasia can lead to cervical carcinoma-in-situ, and eventually cervical cancer.

For the most part, there are no symptoms associated with cervical dysplasia. This is why it's recommended for women to get routine Pap smears, which will show the abnormality and allow for early diagnosis and treatment. An abnormal Pap smear can be seen as soon as a few weeks post-infection, or it can occur many decades after the infection.

Abnormal Pap smears can be a result of inflammation or infections. Some nutritional deficiencies are also linked to abnormal Pap smears. However, the most common cause of an abnormal Pap smear is HPV (human papillomavirus). A new test called the PAPNET, which increases the detection of abnormal cervical cells up to 30 percent, has recently been developed. This FDA-approved test is now available in some medical centers.

The best time to catch and begin treatment for cervical dysplasia is in the beginning stages, before the cells become cancerous. A Pap smear or colposcopy (examination of the cervix and vagina) are the best ways of discovering a problem.

## SUPPLEMENTATION TO TREAT CERVICAL DYSPLASIA

| Supplements | Dosage | Considerations |
|---|---|---|
| Alpha lipoic acid | 100 to 300 milligrams (mg) a day | |
| B-vitamin complex | 50 mg twice a day | Recommended for women taking birth control pills |
| Beta-carotene | 5,000-10,000 international units (IU) | |
| EPA/DHA (fish oil) | 1,000 mg a day | |
| Folate | 400 micrograms twice a day | $B_{12}$ and other B vitamins should be taken while supplementing with folate |
| Lycopene | 10 mg a day | |
| Quercetin | 300 to 900 mg once a day | |
| Rutin | 300 mg once a day | |
| Selenium | 100 to 200 micrograms daily | |
| Zinc | 15 to 25 mg daily | |

## CHOLESTEROL ISSUES

*See* Heart Disease.

## COPPER DEFICIENCY

*See* Osteoporosis.

## CORONARY ARTERY DISEASE

*See* Heart Disease.

## CRAMPS

*See* Premenstrual Syndrome (PMS).

## CYSTIC ACNE

Cystic acne is the most painful type of acne. Some people have constant acne, and others experience occasional or frequent breakouts. People who do not have acne all the time often experience breakouts seven to ten days before their monthly cycle. However, people who suffer from constant acne will notice that it gets worse the week before their cycle.

There are several hormonal imbalances that can cause cystic acne. First, elevated levels of testosterone can cause acne. Consequently, if you have PCOS (see page 122 for more information) you may have an increased risk of developing cycstic acne due to elevated testosterone levels. After menopause, you may also have high testosterone levels that predispose you to breakouts. When you are stressed, increased levels of DHEA can also cause skin lesions. Stress may also cause acne through another mechanism—elevated cortisol levels. With high cortisol levels, your body produces excess oil (which clogs the pores and causes acne) and increases the amount of testosterone that you produce.

Existing acne may get worse at perimenopause when estrogen levels start to decline, resulting in testosterone levels becoming out of balance with the amount of estrogen your body is producing even though your testosterone levels may be normal. When your body makes more estrogen it decreases sebum production, which lowers your risk of developing acne.

## CYSTS

*See* Fibrocystic Breast Disease.

## DEPRESSION

*See* Postpartum Depression; Premenstrual Dysphoric Disorder (PMDD); Premenstrual Syndrome (PMS).

## DIETHYLSTILBESTROL (DES) BABIES

Diethylstilbestrol (DES) is a synthetic, nonsteroidal estrogenic compound first made in the late 1930s. In the 1940s, the FDA approved it for four uses: gonorrheal vaginitis (vaginal inflammation), atrophic vaginitis (which results from lower estrogen levels after menopause, causing the vaginal tissue to become drier and thinner), menopause symptoms, and postpartum lactation suppression. Additionally, physicians formerly gave it to pregnant women to prevent miscarriages. Women were also given DES to try and treat the nausea and vomiting that can occur during pregnancy. Unfortunately, it was not until much later that doctors realized taking DES during pregnancy can lead to an array of negative consequences.

DES has also been used as the "morning after pill."

In the 1970s, some health risks associated with DES came into the light. Some of the effects directly affected the women who took DES. Women prescribed DES while pregnant have a moderately higher risk of developing breast cancer. However, most of the side effects concern the offspring of the women who took DES during pregnancy.

### DES DAUGHTERS

Daughters of mothers who used DES (DES daughters) have an increased risk of developing an abnormal type of vaginal cancer called "adenocarcinoma," a cancer that originates in the glandular tissue. Recent studies have shown that DES can also cause abnormalities in the reproductive tract, immune system, and brain. Additionally, DES daughters have an increased risk of tubal pregnancy (when the fertilized egg implants somewhere other than the uterus), infertility, and premature deliveries.

## ■ Effects of DES on DES Daughters

- Abnormal development of gender-specific sexual behavior (females behave in masculine manners)
- Abnormal estrogen production and receptor function
- Abnormal glucose tolerance, which increases your risk of diabetes
- Abnormal progesterone production and receptor function
- Deformed fallopian tubes and ovaries
- Deformed uteruses that cannot sustain a pregnancy
- Diminished formation of corpora lutea (eggs)
- Elevated levels of prolactin
- Elevated rates of premature babies
- Higher rates of benign and malignant breast tumors
- Higher rates of uterine tumors, both benign and malignant
- Higher than normal infertility rates.
- Immune system dysfunction (changes in the T-helper and natural killer cells)
- Increased frequency of ovarian cysts and abnormal follicles
- Increased rates of ectopic pregnancies (pregnancies when the fertilized egg is implanted outside the uterus) and miscarriages
- Increased rates of endometriosis
- Increased rates of prolactinomas (noncancerous tumors of the pituitary)

## ■ Treatment for DES Daughters

While DES daughters have no control over their exposure to DES, there are some things they can do throughout life to protect their health.

- Conduct a breast self-exam at least once a month.

- Discuss DES with family and especially children. There is not a lot of research on the effects of DES on the children of DES daughters and sons (DES sons will be discussed in the next section), but it is a good idea for them to know about the risks of exposure to DES.

- Schedule regular mammograms and clinical breast examinations. Studies have shown that DES daughters over the age of forty have a greater risk of breast cancer, but younger DES daughters should get checked routinely as well.

- Schedule regular visits to the gynecologist, including Pap smears and pelvic exams. Special precautions during examinations may need to be taken with DES daughters.

- Seek infertility counseling, since many DES daughters have difficulty becoming pregnant.

- Treat all pregnancies as if they are high-risk.

## DES SONS

Sons of mothers who took DES (DES sons) can be affected too. According to studies, DES sons are at a higher risk for epididymal cysts, which are sperm-filled cysts in the epididymis, the tube that lies above and behind each testicle. In her book *It's My Ovaries, Stupid,* Dr. Elizabeth Vliet describes these effects.

### ■ Effects of DES on DES Sons

- Abnormal development of male sexual behavior

- Abnormal glucose tolerance, which increases your risk of diabetes

- Abnormal sperm count and mobility

- Cysts in the epididymis, a part of the male reproductive system

- Higher rate of testicular cancer at earlier than normal ages

- Hypospadius (deformity of the penis)

- Immune system dysfunction

- Increased genital defects

- Low sperm counts

- Reduced fertility

- Stunted testicles and penises

- Undescended testicles

### ■ Treatment for DES Sons

There are a few steps DES Sons can take to protect their health.

- Discuss DES with family and especially children. There is not a lot of research on the effects of DES on the children of DES daughters and sons, but it is a good idea for them to know about the risks of exposure to DES.

- Perform testicular self-exams monthly.

## DIABETES

*See* Heart Disease; Polycystic Ovarian Syndrome (PCOS).

# DYSMENORRHEA

*See* Endometriosis; Premenstrual Syndrome (PMS).

# DYSPAREUNIA

*See* Endometriosis.

# ENDOMETRIOSIS

Endometriosis is a disorder of the female reproductive system. In endometriosis, the cells that form the lining of the uterus (the endometrium) grow outside of the uterus, usually in the abdomen, pelvis, fallopian tubes, or ovaries. However, endometrial tissue can grow anywhere in the body, including the eyes. These areas of tissue growing outside the uterus are called "uterine implants." When you menstruate, the uterine implant bleeds the same way it would if it were inside your uterus: thickening, breaking down, and bleeding. This process sets up an inflammatory condition which is an irritant and causes pain, since there is nowhere for the blood to go. In the United States, between 10 and 15 percent of women between the ages of twenty-four and forty are affected by endometriosis.

The implants also produce their own estrogen by a process called "aromatization." Consequently, even if you take medications to lower your estrogen levels in order to treat the endometriosis, the implant tissue will still produce its own estrogen and cause the surrounding areas to grow. Implants can migrate to your spinal cord and cause intense lower back pain. They can also go into the muscle wall of the uterus, which is called adenomyosis, and cause bleeding into the uterine muscle during your menstrual cycle, causing pain and irritation.

Endometriosis is a state where there is increased aromatase activity. Aromatase is an enzyme that increases the conversion of androgens (like testosterone) to estrogens in the peripheral tissues. With endometriosis, there is also deficient expression of 17-beta-HSD type-2, which impairs inactivation of estradiol (E2) into estrone (E1). Both of these states lead to an increased stimulation of the endometrium and consequent endometriosis.

# Risk Factors for Endometriosis

The main risk factor for endometriosis is family history. If your mother or sister has endometriosis, you are more likely to have it. There is no agreement in the medical community as to the cause of endometriosis, but there are risk factors for developing it.

## ■ Risk Factors for Endometriosis

- Diet low in fruit
- Diet low in green vegetables
- Estrogen dominance
- High intake of red meat
- High-fat diet
- History of abuse
- Immune dysfunction
- Lack of exercise from an early age on
- Menstrual cycles that occur more frequently than every twenty-eight days, with menstrual bleeding lasting more than seven day.
- Naturally red hair
- Use of intrauterine devices (birth control devices placed inside the uterus)

## ■ Possible Risk Factors for Endometriosis*

- Exposure to environmental estrogens or estrogen disruptors (PCBs, weed killers, plastics, detergents, household cleaners, and tin can liners)
- Liver dysfunction
- Long-term exposure to dioxin (a class of toxic chemicals)
- Poor estrogen metabolism
- Prenatal exposure to high levels of estrogen

*Unlike the risk factors in the previous list, which are definite, these are only possible.

As you can see from the list above, consuming or not consuming certain foods is associated with an increased risk of the disease. However, consuming whole grains, liver, milk, carrots, coffee, cheese, or fish were not associated with an increased risk of the disease.

Aromatose activity in the body is increased by being overweight, high cortisol levels, elevated insulin levels, zinc deficiency, inflammation, alcohol consumption, supplementation with the botanical Coleus (Coleus forskohlii), and medications such as isoproterenol. You can decrease your aromatose activity by consuming things like flaxseed, grape seed, and red wine. Vitamin C also helps, and so do some medications, such as Arimidex, ketoconazole, and metformin.

## ■ Causes of Endometriosis

Even though we do not know the cause of endometriosis, some studies have shown that the immune system is involved. Immune markers (blood tests that provide your doctor with information about your immune system) such as IL-8, TNF-alpha, and IL-10 are usually elevated in people who have endometriosis. IL-4 and IFN-gamma, other immune markers, may also be elevated. Women who have endometriosis also have higher rates of autoimmune diseases.

Likewise, diet may also play a role in the etiology of endometriosis. In a study of over 500 women, there was a 40 percent decreased risk of developing endometriosis in those who ate more green vegetables and fresh fruit. Additionally, there was an 80 percent increase in risk of developing endometriosis in those who ate large amounts of red meat.

Environmental toxins may also play a role in the development of endometriosis. Bisphenol-A, parabens, phthalates, pesticides, dioxins, PCBs, solvents, and fomaldehyde have all been implicated. New testing methods are now available to measure many of these levels in your body by Metametrix Clinical Laboratory (see page 184). Many women are exposed to environmental toxins, but not all of them develop endometriosis. Some women have a genetic single nucleotide polymorphism (SNP) that increases their risk of developing endometriosis when they are exposed to these products. Studies have shown that women with a polymorphism of the cytochrome P450 1A1 gene and the glutathione S-transferase M1 gene have an increased risk of developing endometriosis.

## ■ Symptoms of Endometriosis

Symptoms of endometriosis vary. The pain you experience may not correlate with the extent of the disease. You can have large areas of endometriosis and little pain, or you can have only a few areas of endometriosis and a great deal of pain. The amount of pain seems to be determined by the depth of the lesions of endometriosis as opposed to the amount of tissue involved.

There are a few main symptoms that you may have with endometriosis:

- ☐ Excessive bleeding during or between periods
- ☐ Infertility
- ☐ Painful intercourse (dyspareunia)
- ☐ Painful menstrual cycles (dysmenorrhea)
- ☐ Pelvic pain

Pain associated with endometriosis may occur not only during the menstrual cycle, but for one or two days before as well. If you are experiencing pelvic pain, it may bother you for the entire month.

Endometriosis is also associated with some less common symptoms:

- ☐ Back pain that radiates down the legs
- ☐ Blood in the bowels, nose, or eyes
- ☐ Diarrhea
- ☐ Fainting
- ☐ Fatigue
- ☐ Pain during urination
- ☐ Painful bowel movements
- ☐ Vomiting

When endometrial tissue forms outside the uterus, free radicals—which are molecules that lack an electron—can also be produced. This causes inflammation.

Women with endometriosis have been found to suppress natural killer cell (NK cell) levels in the peritoneal fluid, the fluid that lines the abdominal wall. NK cells are produced by the body as part of the immune system in response to an "invasion" of abnormal cells or tissue. Low NK cell levels may consequently be part of the reason the body does not destroy the endometrial implants. Additionally, women with endometriosis may have high IgG and IgM (immunoglobulin) levels. Sometimes, sufferers produce antibodies against their ovaries and endometrial cells. Both abnormal levels of immunoglobulins and antibodies set up a process were the body literally starts attacking itself. This is called an autoimmune reaction.

## Treating Endometriosis

Treatment frequently centers around hormonal balance. Conventionally, in medicine, this is done with oral contraceptives which usually contain both estrogen and progesterone. However, since the hormonal imbalance associated with endometriosis seems to be due to estrogen excess, taking natural progesterone by itself is very advantageous.

Progesterone can modify the action of E2, thus decreasing the amount of time estrogen stays on its receptor sites. This will decrease the amount of circulating estrogen. Progesterone is also helpful since it can decrease the amount of uterine contractions that can occur with endometriosis. Uterine contractions are one of the causes of pain in patients who have endometriosis.

Some women who have endometriosis do not have estrogen excess. As was previously stated, uterine implants can make their own estrogen. If this happens, the remainder of the body may have low estrogen levels. If you have decreased estrogen levels, you will have symptoms of low estrogen, even if you are not peri- or postmenopausal. This is why it is very important to have your hormone levels measured. A twenty-eight-day salivary test (with samples taken eleven of the twenty-eight days)

## DIAGNOSING ENDOMETRIOSIS

During a physical examination, your healthcare practitioner may find tenderness in your pelvis if you have endometriosis. There are a few ways to detect this:

- Blood test. Women who suffer from the disease have certain proteins in their blood that can be detected by a cancer antigen 125 blood test.

- Pelvic exam. During a pelvic exam, your doctor manually feels your pelvis for abnormalities.

- Ultrasounds. Ultrasounds can be helpful in detecting endometriosis. They use scanners and sound waves to provide a video image of your reproductive organs.

However, the only definitive way to diagnose endometriosis is made by laparoscopy, which is when the doctor looks inside your abdomen and takes a biopsy specimen. A laparoscope (a viewing instrument) is inserted into the abdomen via a tiny incision. It allows the doctor to view the abdomen and its surrounding areas. This test can detect the location and the size of the endometriosis.

would be the best way to determine exactly which hormones are low and which are high if you have endometriosis.

There are other treatments for endometriosis that have been shown to be beneficial. Diet and nutrition are very important.

- Botanical medicines are very advantageous if you have endometriosis. For example, dandelion root (taraxacum officinale) is a wonderful herb that helps detoxify the liver and gallbladder, which consequently helps detoxify estrogen. Dandelion leaf is also helpful because it contains vitamins A, C, and K; calcium; and choline. Leonorus (motherwort) is another botanical agent that decreases spasms and soothes the nerves. Motherwort helps decrease pain and is also a mild sedative.

- Caffeine consumption has been negatively linked to endometriosis. A study showed that women who consume high amounts of caffeine (5 to 7 grams per month) have a 1.2 times greater risk of developing endometriosis. Women who consume more than 7 grams a month have a 1.6 times greater risk.

- Consuming onions, garlic, and leeks, which all contain sulfur (a non-metallic element that enhances your immune system) will also help.

- A diet that is low in animal protein also aids the body in detoxification and decreases inflammation.

- Foods that are high in fiber help the body eliminate metabolic wastes.

- Increasing your intake of vegetables effectively helps your liver metabolize estrogen properly and also aids in the elimination of toxins. Broccoli, Brussels sprouts, cauliflower, cabbage, kale, and other vegetables that contain indole-3-carbinol help the body metabolize estrogen. Other foods that help cleanse your liver are carrots, lemons, artichokes, beets, watercress, and dandelion greens.

- Prickly ash (xanthoxylum americanum) has a beneficial action on capillary engorgement and sluggish circulation. It stimulates blood flow and increases the transport of oxygen and nutrients along with removing cellular waste products. If you have endometriosis, prickly ash is valuable to enhance circulation throughout the pelvis.

- Seaweed helps to stimulate T-cell production, which enhances your immune system. T-cells are a type of white blood cell that helps the body's immune system defend against diseases.

- Some herbs and spices decrease inflammation. Additionally, the same herbs that are helpful for menstrual cramps are useful if you experience pain with endometriosis. Valerian, crampbark, black cohosh, wild yam, chamomile, blue cohash, ginger, passion flower, and false unicorn root will all do the trick. Chaste tree (vitex agnus castus) increases progesterone production by increasing luteinzing hormone. With its use, estrogen is less available to stimulate the tissue of the endometrium.

- Taking good bacteria (probiotics) may be helpful. Your body needs good bacteria in its intestinal tract in order to break down estrogen. Probiotics are available in pill or powder form.

- Turska's formula is a tincture formula that can be used if you have endometriosis. Tincture formulas are liquid mixtures of herbal extracts formulated for specific needs. Turska's formula contains Aconite napellus (monkshood), Gelsemium sempervirens (Yellow Jasmine), Bryonia alba (Bryony), and Phytolacca Americana (Poke Root). These botanicals may interfere with the placement of the lesions that occur in endometriosis and enhance the immune system. Turska's formula is only available through a healthcare practitioner.

## OTHER SUPPLEMENTATION TO TREAT ENDOMETRIOSIS

| Supplements | Dosage | Considerations |
| --- | --- | --- |
| Alpha-linolenic acid | 500 to 1,000 mg | Contained in flax seed, canola, pumpkin, soy, and walnuts. |
| B-vitamins | B complex 100 mg | Detoxify estrogen. Take twice a day since they dissolve the same day they are ingested, and always take a multivitamin that contains B-vitamins. |
| Beta-carotene (a type of vitamin A) | 5,000 IU | Aids the immune system and increases T-cell levels. |
| Omega-3 fatty acids | 1,000 to 2,000 mg | Contained in EPA, DHA, fish oil, fish, lamb, and nuts. |
| Omega-6 fatty acids | 500 to 1,000 mg | Contained in borage, black current, and evening primrose oil. |
| Pycnogenol | 30 mg twice a day | Taking this supplement in the given amount for six months has been shown to significantly reduce pain from endometriosis. |

| Selenium | 50 to 200 micrograms | Aids thyroid function and the immune system, and reduces heavy metal toxicity in the blood. |
| --- | --- | --- |
| Vitamin C | 1,000 mg | Helps enhance immune system, and decreases autoimmune production, capillary fragility, and fatigue. |
| Vitamin E | 400 IU | Helps correct estrogen/progesterone ratio. |

# FATIGUE

See Endometriosis; Postpartum Depression; Premenstrual Dysphoric Disorder (PMDD); Premenstrual Syndrome (PMS).

# FIBROCYSTIC BREAST DISEASE

Fibrocystic breast disease is a condition where there are noncancerous changes, or cysts, in the tissues of the breasts. These changes can cause pain and discomfort. It is estimated that over 60 percent of women will be affected by fibrocystic breast disease in their lifetime.

## ■ Symptoms of Fibrocystic Breast Disease

The symptoms associated with the disease vary in severity. Generally, they are at their worst before each period.

☐ Bumpy consistency in breast tissue (usually the outer part of the breast)

☐ Feeling of discomfort in breasts

☐ Occasional nipple discharge (which always needs to be evaluated by a physician)

☐ Premenstrual tenderness and swelling of the breasts

### DIAGNOSING FIBROCYSTIC BREAST DISEASE

There are a few ways to test for fibrocystic breast disease. Healthcare providers can perform a breast exam, which would reveal masses in the tissue. Mammograms, which are low-dose x-rays used to examine breasts, are also useful. Breast ultrasounds are also helpful, but sometimes a biopsy of the breast is necessary.

## ■ Causes of Fibrocystic Breast Disease

All of the causes of fibrocystic breast disease are not completely known. However, the following list contains items believed to cause or contribute to the disease:

- Caffeine consumption
- Estrogen dominance
- Family history
- High-fat diet
- Iodine deficiency

## ■ Treating Fibrocystic Breast Disease

- Elimination of caffeine from your diet.
- Iodine replacement with iodine/ iodide. (You should have your iodine levels measured before starting supplementation. This is a twenty-four-hour urine test.)
- Limiting the intake of "bad" fats.
- Performing a monthly self-examination of breasts.
- Progesterone replacement.

# FIBROIDS

Fibroids, which are known as *leiomyomata*, are benign (non-cancerous) growths on or within the walls of the uterus. These tumors can be a variety of different sizes and quantities. The resulting symptoms depend upon these factors. If the fibroids are small and do not cause any symptoms, a doctor may recommend that no course of action be taken. However, larger—or multiple—fibroids can cause pain, excessive bleeding, and problems urinating, as well as infertility and premature labor. When fibroids cause serious problems such as these, treatment options include surgery (hysterectomy or myomectomy), medications (such as oral contraceptives), and procedures such as the high-intensity focused ultrasound (which uses ultrasound waves to destroy the fibroid tissue). Although no substitute for necessary surgery or other medical action, the nutrients in the table on page 90 may allow these procedures to be avoided by shrinking the uterine fibroids naturally. You should also avoid drinking coffee.

Fibroids have estrogen receptors, and are thus responsive to the body's level of estrogen. During periods of pregnancy, when estrogen levels increase, fibroids tend to grow in size. After menopause, on the other hand, when estrogen levels drop significantly, fibroids usually become smaller. For this reason, doctors will often recommend a medication with an estrogen-lowering effect, which will artificially create this situation. Similarly, you may find it effective to take natural progesterone, which directly effects the estrogen in your body. Your doctor will be able to prescribe a specific daily dosage.

| SUPPLEMENTATION TO TREAT FIBROIDS | | |
|---|---|---|
| Supplements | Dosage | Considerations |
| Alpha lipoic acid | 300 mg once a day | Improves blood sugar levels so diabetics may be able to take less medication. |
| Carnitine | 1,500 mg once a day | |
| Coenzyme Q-10 | 100 mg once a day | May reduce the effects of blood thinners. Doses over 100 mg may cause diarrhea. |
| Gamma-linolenic acid (GLA) | 240 to 720 mg once a day | It is important to maintain the proper ratio of omega-6 fatty acids to omega-3 fatty acids. |
| Inositol | 500 mg twice a day | May stimulate uterine contractions. Women who wish to become pregnant should consult their doctors regarding its use. |
| Magnesium | 400 mg once a day | Consult healthcare provider for dosage if you have kidney disease. Discontinue use and see your doctor if you experience abdominal pain. Take a lower dose if it causes diarrhea. |
| Milk thistle | 100 to 200 mg once a day | Reduces efficiency of certain blood pressure medications. |
| Phosphatidylcholine (Lecithin) | 2,000 mg once a day | Use with caution if you have malabsorption problems, as this could exacerbate them. |

# FOOD CRAVINGS

*See* Premenstrual Syndrome (PMS).

# HEADACHES

*See* Migraines; Premenstrual Dysphoric Disorder (PMDD); Premenstrual Syndrome (PMS).

# HEART ATTACK

*See* Heart Disease.

# HEART DISEASE

Heart disease is not a specific disease, but rather a broad term used to describe a number of diseases that can affect your heart and, in some cases, your blood vessels. Heart disease is also called cardiovascular disease, and can include coronary artery disease, arrhythmias, blocked vessels that can lead to heart attacks or stroke, heart infections, and heart defects you are born with.

Heart disease is the number one killer of men and women worldwide. Therefore, it is important to do all you can to prevent and treat heart disease before it affects you and your loved ones. To do this, you need to know what the risk factors for heart disease are.

Many people think that if they watch their cholesterol, they will drastically reduce their risk of developing heart disease. However, cholesterol is only part of the picture—one-half of women who die of heart disease have normal cholesterol levels. There are quite a few other risk factors that have to do with hormones and menopause that women should pay attention to.

## OTHER RISK FACTORS FOR HEART DISEASE

It is important that as a woman you have your other risk factors (besides cholesterol) of heart disease measured. The risk factors you need to look out for are homocysteine, iron (ferritin), lipoprotein A, fibrinogen, and C-reactive protein. Finally, there is a test that checks for more than a standard cholesterol test does. This is called the vertical auto profile (VAP) test. This test may also be called an LPP test. This test is a more accurate way of measuring LDL (bad cholesterol) since it is a direct measure of LDL. A cholesterol panel gives you a calculated measurement. A VAP (or LPP) test also allows measurement of the lipoprotein subclasses of HDL and LDL. These include HDL-2, HDL-3, intermediate-density lipoprotein (IDL), and very-low-density lipoproteins (VLDL-1, VLDL-2, and VLDL-3). These subclasses examine particle size. If the particle size of cholesterol is small it is more of a risk factor for heart disease than if the particle size

# Primary Risk Factors for Heart Disease

Along with cholesterol, some common risk factors for heart disease are:

- Age. The older you are, the higher your risk of developing heart disease.

- Blood pressure. High blood pressure (hypertension) increases your chance of developing heart disease.

- Diabetes. Diabetics have a greater risk of developing heart disease.

- Diet. A diet high in fat, salt, or cholesterol can increase your chances of getting heart disease.

- Gender. Men are usually at a higher risk of developing heart disease than women, until after menopause when women have as high or higher risk of developing the disease.

- Genetics. Having heart disease in your family increases your chances of developing the disease.

- Hygiene. Poor oral hygiene can lead to infections, which can worsen your risk of developing heart disease.

- Lack of exercise. Not exercising increases your risk of developing heart disease.

- Obesity. Excess weight increases your chances of developing the disease.

- Smoking. Smoking increases your chances of developing the disease.

- Stress. Unresolved stress can damage arteries and worsen other risk factors.

is large. For example, you can have a high HDL (good cholesterol) level but if the particle size of HDL is mostly small, then your risk for developing heart disease is still increased.

## Homocysteine

Homocysteine is an amino acid produced by ineffective protein metabolism that promotes free radical production. Free radicals are molecules that lack an electron. They will search through your body for an electron until they find a healthy cell, and then they steal the healthy cell's electron. This process kills the cell. If enough cells die, then you expire. This process is also one of the causes of oxidative stress, which can lead to vascular disease, a condition that affects your circulatory system. Oxidative stress is a term used to describe internal inflammation and the free radicals produced as a result of this inflammation. It is caused by an imbalance between the production of reactive oxygen and the body's ability to detoxify it.

Elevated homocysteine levels can greatly increase your chances of developing heart disease. Additionally, your homocysteine levels may naturally increase with menopause, so it's good to get your levels checked regularly at that age.

High homocysteine levels can damage the arterial lining of the heart, making it narrow and inelastic (a condition also known as "hardening" of the arteries, or arteriosclerosis). When levels are elevated, homocysteine can reduce nitric oxide production, which can lead to high blood pressure, a risk factor for heart disease. High homocysteine levels also elevate triglyceride and cholesterol synthesis.

Studies suggest that 42 percent of strokes, 28 percent of peripheral vascular disease (which causes leg pain, cramping, and loss of circulation), and approximately 30 percent of cardiovascular disease (heart attacks, chest pain) are directly related to elevated homocysteine levels. Furthermore, a study published in the *New England Journal of Medicine* in July 1997 showed that people with homocysteine levels below nine were much less likely to die. Optimal levels of homocysteine are six to eight. Another study showed that women with a history of high blood pressure and elevated homocysteine levels were 25 times more likely to have a heart attack or stroke than women whose blood pressure and homocysteine levels were closer to normal.

## ■ Causes of Excess Homocysteine

- Drugs
- Hereditary predisposition
- Hypothyroidism
- Menopause
- Renal failure
- Smoking
- Toxins

In instances where high homocysteine levels are hereditary, it is usually due to the fact that some people are lacking the enzyme methylenetetrahydrofolate reductase, which breaks down homocysteine. A deficiency of this enzyme increases the need for folate in order to prevent high homocysteine levels. This occurs in 12 percent of the population.

Elevated homocysteine levels have also been associated with several other disease processes including depression, osteoporosis, multiple sclerosis (MS), spina bifida/neural tube defects, spontaneous abortion, placental abruption, type-2 diabetes, renal failure, and rheumatoid arthritis. Additionally, elevated homocysteine levels have recently been associated with the risk of memory loss later in life and an increase in breast cancer risk.

As mentioned, your homocysteine levels are lower before menopause. As you go through menopause, your homocysteine levels will rise because your lowering estrogen status is associated with elevated homocysteine concentrations.

## ■ Ways to Lower Homocysteine Levels

- Exercise
- Hormone replacement therapy, specifically with estrogen
- Stress reduction
- Supplementation with vitamins $B_6$, $B_{12}$, and folate

As previously stated, your body needs adequate amounts of $B_6$, $B_{12}$, and folate in order to break down homocysteine. B vitamins are water soluble and excessive ingestion of caffeine products, alcohol, or diuretics (water pills) will wash B vitamins out of your system. Some people may still have elevated homocysteine levels after supplementing with $B_6$, $B_{12}$, and folate. These people will need to take the active form of folic acid (L-5-MTHF).

Researchers have suggested that folate supplementation could save 20,000 to 50,000 lives from heart disease every year. In addition to supplementation, folate can be found in dark green leafy vegetables, beans, legumes, and oranges.

Consuming broccoli, spinach, and beets also increase the conversion of homocysteine in your body. Likewise, SAM-e (s-adenosylmethionine) will also help break down homocysteine. The suggested dosage is 200 to 400 mg a day.

Garlic at the dosage of 1,000 mg a day and trimethylglycine at 500 to 1,000 mg a day have also been found to lower homocysteine levels.

## Iron

When women menstruate, many of them are instructed by medical professionals to take iron supplementation, because blood loss sometimes results in low iron levels, or in some cases, anemia. Consequently, when you go through menopause, you are no longer menstruating, so there is a good chance that if you once needed iron supplementation, you will no longer need it after menopause.

In many cases, if you continue with iron supplementation after menopause, your iron levels will become too high. Studies have shown that too much iron can increase your risk of heart disease. Every 1 percent increase in ferritin (serum iron) causes a 4 percent elevation in risk of heart attack. Thus, continuing iron supplementation if you do not need it may elevate your ferritin level and predispose you to a heart attack. Also, your levels of iron increase naturally after menopause since you are no longer bleeding every month, so it is a good idea to have your ferritin (iron) levels measured.

## Lipoprotein (a)

For the most part, elevated lipoprotein (a) levels are inherited. However, like many of the other risk factors for heart disease discussed, lipoprotein (a) levels also increase naturally after menopause and can increase your risk of developing heart disease. Also, statin drugs, which are used to lower cholesterol, have been shown to increase lipoprotein (a) levels.

Lipoprotein (a) is a small cholesterol particle that causes inflammation and can clog your blood vessels. Research has shown that people with elevated lipoprotein (a) have a 70 percent higher risk of developing heart disease over ten years.

Lipoprotein (a) regulates clot formation and decreases blood thinning. If your blood becomes too thick you have an increased risk of heart attack and stroke. This process is increased in diabetes and in menopause.

There are some ways you can lower your lipoprotein (a) levels, should they become too high. If you plan to use any of these methods to reduce your levels, be sure to do them daily. You should work with a physician who is familiar with treating high lipoprotein (a) levels to determine which treatment is right for you.

### ■ Ways to Lower Lipoprotein (a) Levels

- Coenzyme Q-10 (120 mg)
- DHA (1 to 2 g)
- Flax seed
- L-carnitine (1 to 2 grams)
- L-lysine (500 to 1,000 mg)
- L-proline (500 to 1,000 mg)
- Nattokinase (50 to 100 mg)*

- Natural estrogen replacement (you should have your levels measured to determine how much estrogen you need).
- Niacin (1 to 2 grams). Do not take if you have insulin resistance or diabetes.
- Vitamin C (2 to 4 g)

*Cannot take if you are on Coumadin, a blood thinner.*

## Fibrinogen

Fibrinogen is a clot-promoting substance in your blood. If the blood levels of fibrinogen are too high, it can cause a heart attack. During menopause, estrogen levels decline. Fibrinogen increases as estrogen decreases, so when you become menopausal, your fibrinogen levels can elevate. Additionally, fibrinogen also elevates if you are a smoker.

Research has shown that estrogen replacement therapy can decrease fibrinogen. Nutritional support includes garlic, coldwater fish, vitamin E, ginkgo, and bromelain. All of these substances can offset the clotting effects of fibrinogen.

## C-reactive Protein

Scientists believe that some infections can cause heart disease. Chlamydia, herpes, and cytomegalovirus, an infection in the herpes group, can cause inflammation in your blood vessels and cause plaque formation, eventually leading to heart disease. Chronic gum disease and an H. pylori infection in your stomach are also causes of inflammation. Elevated levels of C-reactive protein (CRP) occur when there is inflammation in the body. High levels are a risk factor for heart disease, diabetes, and hypertension. Since CRP levels can be elevated due to many causes of inflammation, your doctor will want to get a high-sensitivity CRP test, which is designed for greater accuracy in measuring risk factors for cardiovascular disease. Studies have shown that C-reactive protein can be predictive of future heart attacks, even if you have a normal cholesterol level. Many physicians believe that an elevated CRP level is the most important risk factor for heart disease.

### ■ Ways to Lower C-Reactive Protein Levels

- Baby aspirin, one per day (check with your doctor first)
- Coenzyme Q-10
- Curcumin (200 to 600 mg per day)
- Essential fatty acids, such as EPA/DHA or fish oil (1,000 mg per day)
- Exercise
- Grapeseed extract (100 to 200 mg per day)
- Green tea (3 cups per day)
- Natural COX-2 inhibitors
- Quercetin supplementation*
- Rosemary
- Statin drugs used to lower cholesterol

* Also found in apples, black tea, and onions.

## HEAVY PERIODS

*See* Endometriosis.

## HIGH BLOOD PRESSURE

*See* Heart Disease; Polycystic Ovarian Syndrome (PCOS).

## HOT FLASHES

*See* Menopause; Premature Ovarian Decline (POD); Premenstrual Syndrome (PMS).

## HUMAN PAPILLOMAVIRUS (HPV)

*See* Cervical Dysplasia (Abnormal Pap Smear).

## HYPERTENSION

*See* Heart Disease; Polycystic Ovarian Syndrome (PCOS).

## HYPOGLYCEMIA

*See* Premenstrual Syndrome (PMS).

## HYSTERECTOMY

*See* Menopause.

## INCONTINENCE

*See* Bladder Problems.

## INFLAMMATION

*See* Endometriosis; Skin Problems.

## INSOMNIA

*See* Postpartum Depression; Premenstrual Dysphoric Disorder (PMDD); Premenstrual Syndrome (PMS).

## IRON TOXICITY

*See* Heart Disease.

## IRREGULAR MENSTRUAL CYCLES

*See* Menopause; Polycystic Ovarian Syndrome (PCOS); Premature Ovarian Decline (POD).

## IRRITABILITY

*See* Menopause; Postpartum Depression; Premature Ovarian Decline (POD); Premenstrual Dysphoric Disorder (PMDD).

## KIDNEY FAILURE

*See* Heart Disease.

## LOW BLOOD SUGAR

*See* Premenstrual Syndrome (PMS).

## MAGNESIUM DEFICIENCY

*See* Osteoporosis.

# MALNUTRITION

*See* Premature Ovarian Decline (POD).

# MENOPAUSE

Every day in the United States, 3,500 women enter menopause. Menopause is defined as the permanent end of menstruation and fertility. It may just be the best time in a woman's life. You no longer have to worry about an unwanted pregnancy, your responsibilities of child rearing are gone, and you are still young and sexually interested. Menopause is a time you get to focus on yourself. Prior to this time, you have likely been busy taking care of other people. Now, "middle-age" begins at the age of sixty.

Menopause occurs naturally in women when the ovaries begin making less estrogen and progesterone. However, if your hormonal symphony is out of tune, you can begin to have symptoms of menopause as early as fifteen years prior to actual menopause.

The time just before menopause in your life is called perimenopause. This is the time when your body begins its transition into menopause, usually starting anywhere from two to eight years before menopause and lasting up until the first year after your final period. Your estrogen levels rise and fall unevenly during this time. You may still have menstrual cycles during perimenpause, but they might become more irregular. Also, the amount that you bleed during each cycle may be more or less than you previously experienced.

The average age to go through menopause ranges from thirty-five to fifty-five. Therefore, you may easily live one-half of your life without a menstrual cycle.

## DIAGNOSING MENOPAUSE

The diagnosis of menopause is made by your physician when you have had no cycle for one year and your blood levels of FSH and LH are elevated.

## ■ Symptoms of Perimenopause and Menopause

- ☐ Aching ankles, knees, wrists, shoulders, and heels
- ☐ Bloating
- ☐ Decreased sexual interest*
- ☐ Depression
- ☐ Dizzy spells
- ☐ Flatulence (gas)
- ☐ Frequent urination
- ☐ Hair growth on face
- ☐ Hair loss
- ☐ Hot flashes
- ☐ Indigestion
- ☐ Insomnia
- ☐ Irritability
- ☐ Lower back pain
- ☐ Memory lapses, lack of focus/ concentration
- ☐ Migraine headaches
- ☐ Mood swings
- ☐ Night sweats
- ☐ Osteoporosis or osteopenia
- ☐ Painful intercourse
- ☐ Palpitations
- ☐ Panic attacks
- ☐ Skin feeling crawly
- ☐ Snoring
- ☐ Sore breasts
- ☐ Urinary leakage
- ☐ Urinary tract infections
- ☐ Vaginal dryness
- ☐ Vaginal itching
- ☐ Vaginal odor
- ☐ Varicose veins
- ☐ Weight gain
- ☐ Weird dreams

* *Loss of sexual interest can occur at menopause, but this is not really a "normal" finding if DHEA continues to make estrogen and testosterone after menopause. However, if DHEA is not making these hormones at sufficient levels, sexual interest can be decreased. Sexual interest may also be lower due to lack of progesterone if you are not sleeping well. Furthermore, abnormal cortisol levels can cause sexual interest to decline.*

## WEIGHT GAIN AND MENOPAUSE

Most women gain weight during menopause. This is due to an imbalance of hormones.

It is the ratio of ovarian hormones that determines how much weight you will gain and where you will gain it. For example, if estradiol (E2) decreases and progesterone, testosterone, and DHEA are normal, then you may gain fat around the middle. Or, if the ratio of E2 to progesterone is high, you may gain weight around the hips.

Progesterone increases fat storage and decreases sensitivity to insulin. Therefore, if you only replace progesterone during menopause and you are also estrogen-deficient, you can predispose yourself to weight gain and diabetes.

Cortisol, one of your sex hormones, facilitates the storage of body fat. If cortisol levels increase, you will store more fat, increase muscle breakdown, and increase insulin resistance. If your cortisol levels remain high, your body goes into the "flight or fight" response, and you gain weight. (For more on this subject, see the section on cortisol on page 32.)

### ■ Additional Facts About Hormones and Weight Gain

- Women who take HRT and are hormonally balanced gain less weight than those who don't.

- Prolonged stress can decrease the function of the ovaries and hormone production, which can also cause weight gain.

- Obesity leads to higher levels of estrone (E1), the estrogen associated with an increase in breast cancer risk.

## TREATING MENOPAUSE

The treatment you need at menopause is as individualized as is your own fingerprint. The goal is to not only alleviate symptoms but to also prevent disease. Make sure that you see a fellowship-trained practitioner in Metabolic/Anti-Aging Medicine who also has a Master's Degree in Metabolic and Nutritional Medicine.

For women who are still cycling, progesterone is usually given days twelve to twenty-four of the cycle. For postmenopausal women, low dose hormones are recommended. Doses that are low help you maintain vision, memory, and mobility, and also help alleviate symptoms commonly associated with menopause. There is really not a reason postmenopausally to use high dose hormones. If you choose to, then you must cycle. If you use low dose hormonal therapy, then the choice to cycle or not is up to you.

## Risk Factors for Perimenopause and Menopause

Generally, menopause occurs naturally. However, certain treatments can speed up the process. For example, a partial or total hysterectomy (sometimes called surgical menopause) can cause menopause to occur earlier than anticipated. Chemotherapy and radiation therapy can have similar effects. Additionally, women who suffer from premature ovarian failure (POF) sometimes experience menopause at earlier ages. (For more on POF, see the section on premature ovarian decline, starting on page 131.)

Most commonly, physicians and other healthcare practitioners recommend that for the first year of menopause—while you are trying to balance all of your hormonal levels—you take the medications daily. After the first year or two, your symptoms will likely have improved. In this case, most healthcare practitioners recommend a hormonal holiday. This can be done by taking all of your hormones days one to twenty-four and no hormones on days twenty-five to twenty-eight. If your hormones are balanced when you do this, you will not have a cycle.

However, many women describe that their memory is not as sharp when they do not take their hormones for a couple of days. Consequently, most postmenopausal women take their prescription hormone replacement Monday through Saturday, taking no hormones on Sunday. This still gives you a weekly hormonal holiday during the month.

## SURGICAL MENOPAUSE

Surgical menopause is the removal of the ovaries in women who haven't yet experienced natural menopause. It almost always occurs with a hysterectomy, which is the removal of the uterus.

One-third of women in the United States have had a hysterectomy. The average age for this operation is thirty-five. Women who have had a partial hysterectomy, which is when the ovaries are left in, can still have a change in hormonal function. Research has shown that about 60 to 70 percent of women experience a decrease in hormones (to menopausal levels) within three to four years of the operation. For some women, progesterone levels may fall within several months of the surgery and estrogen levels may decline within one to two years. The changes in hormone levels occur because your uterine artery is cut and tied off during the hysterectomy, which decreases blood flow to your ovaries. Surgical menopause reduces testosterone levels to a greater degree than natural menopause does.

## MIGRAINES

Migraines are severe, painful headaches with often disabling symptoms. Many women who get migraine headaches suffer from ones that are hormonally related. Some women get headaches when their estrogen and/or progesterone levels drop just before the start of their cycle. At ovulation, estrogen levels drop and progesterone levels elevate. This causes some women to get migraine headaches. Additionally, the fluctuating levels of estrogen at perimenopause may cause migraine headaches in women who have never had them, or increase the intensity and frequency of headaches in women who already suffer from hormonally-related headaches.

Estrogen levels affect headaches in several ways.

- Declining estrogen can cause vasoconstriction, which is when the muscles in the walls of the arteries become tighter, which increases migraine pain.

- Declining estrogen levels lower women's pain threshold, which makes nerve endings more sensitive to pain-causing stimuli.

- Decreasing estrogen levels cause an increase in norepinephrine (NE) in the brain, a neurotransmitter that enhances vasoconstriction (constriction of the vessel) and decreases blood flow to the parts of the brain that can produce an aura experienced by many migraine suffers. This also intensifies the pain from the migraine headache.

- Decreasing estrogen levels can lower beta-endorphins, which help relieve pain.

- Falling estrogen levels can cause a rebound in dopamine, which can increase pain.

- Lower estrogen levels decrease serotonin levels at serotonin receptor sites, which are paramount in decreasing migraine pain. When serotonin levels fall, blood vessels in the brain can spasm. If this occurs, the result may be a migraine headache. Even worse, a blood vessel spasm can be a causative factor for a stroke.

Augmenting progesterone on days twenty-two to twenty-five of the menstrual cycle will ensure that the drop in progesterone is not so abrupt. This helps many women decrease the severity and number of menstrually-related migraine headaches. Synthetic progesterone (progestin) in birth control pills can increase the frequency and severity of migraine headaches that are both hormonally and non-hormonally related. Supplementing with coenzyme Q-10 (200 to 300 mg a day) along with taking extra magnesium has also been found to be helpful in the prevention and treatment of menstrual migraines.

## MOOD SWINGS

*See* Menopausse; Postpartum Depression; Premenstrual Dysphoric Disorder (PMDD); Premenstrual Syndrome (PMS).

## NAUSEA

*See* Premenstrual Syndrome (PMS).

## NIGHT SWEATS

*See* Menopause; Premature Ovarian Decline (POD).

## OBESITY

*See* Heart Disease.

## OSTEOPENIA

*See* Osteoporosis.

## OSTEOPOROSIS

Osteoporosis is a disease in which bones become more fragile and more likely to break. If untreated, the disease can progress painlessly until a bone breaks. The most common places people with osteoporosis experience fractures are the hip, the spine, and the wrists. Mild bone loss is called osteopenia. Major bone loss is called osteoporosis.

In North America, Europe, Australia, and Asia, it is estimated that one in every three women fifty-five years old or older will have a fracture from osteoporosis. Globally, about 1.7 billion hip fractures occur each year. Of the women who break a hip, half will never walk again. This number is expected to increase four-fold by 2050 with the greatest increases expected in Africa and Asia. In the United States, almost half of women over sixty have osteoporosis.

Bone mineral density is not enough. The strength of bone is also important. Almost 50 percent of bone fractures occur in people who have normal bone density.

## ■ Symptoms of Osteoporosis

☐ Back pain                     ☐ Bone fractures                     ☐ Loss of height

# CAUSES AND TREATMENT FOR OSTEOPOROSIS

Bones are constantly breaking down and reforming, reabsorbing and depositing calcium as this occurs. As people age, the ratio of breakdown and reformation changes, with bone breakdown eventually exceeding bone formation. This change in ratio is higher in postmenopausal women.

To maintain your bone health, your body needs calcium, magnesium, boron, zinc, copper, silicon, phosphorus, manganese, vitamins $B_6$, $B_{12}$, D, and K, folate, and strontium. Additionally, your body has to have an optimal amount of bioflavones and amino acids to maintain and build bone.

## Calcium

Calcium is the most abundant mineral in the body. More than 99 percent of the body's calcium is in its bones and teeth. Calcium has many functions in the body, including the important role it plays in supporting bone and tooth structure. Calcium reduces bone loss and decreases bone turnover. Numerous studies have shown that calcium supplementation can help decrease bone loss by 30 to 50 percent.

## ■ Important Facts About Calcium

- Calcium carbonate is not the best form of calcium to use. Calcium citrate or hydroxyappetite are now the preferred forms.

- Calcium intake helps lower cholesterol.

- Calcium is also needed for the absorption of vitamin $B_{12}$.

- Calcium should be taken throughout the day for maximum absorption, because your body can only absorb 500 mg at a time. It is best taken with meals and at bed time.

- Consuming Tums is not a good way to intake calcium, due to poor absorption.

- Hydrochloric acid, citric acid, glycine, and lysine all help increase calcium absorption.

- Milk is not the best source of calcium since pasteurization destroys up to 32 percent of the available calcium.

- Use only pharmaceutical grade calcium supplements. Lower grade products may be contaminated with lead, mercury, arsenic, aluminum, or cadmium. (For suggestions on companies that use pharmaceutical grade supplements see the Resources section on page 183.)

- Vitamin C increases calcium absorption by 100 percent.

- You can take too much calcium.

Besides supplementation, there are many foods you can eat to get calcium.

### ▧ Food Sources of Calcium

| | | |
|---|---|---|
| • Almonds | • English walnuts | • Prunes, dried |
| • Barley | • Garbanzo beans | • Rice, brown |
| • Beet greens | • Ground beef | • Salmon |
| • Black beans | • Halibut | • Sesame seeds |
| • Bluefish | • Hazelnuts | • Shrimp |
| • Brazil nuts | • Kale | • Soybeans |
| • Brick cheese | • Kelp | • Sunflower seeds |
| • Broccoli | • Mackerel | • Tofu |
| • Chicken | • Mustard greens | • Turnip greens |
| • Chinese cabbage | • Olives, ripe | • Watercress |
| • Dandelion greens | • Parsley | • White beans |
| • Dates | • Pecans | • Yogurt |
| • Eggs | • Pinto beans | |

When you're looking to increase your calcium, there are a few things you should avoid. The items on the following list all decrease calcium absorption.

## ■ Factors That Decrease Calcium Absorption

- Acidic foods
- Alcohol
- Aspartame
- Aspirin
- Beer
- Blueberry
- Caffeine
- Certain medications:
  Cholestyramine
  Excessive thyroid
    replacement
  *Heparin*
  Methotrexate
  Phenobarbital
  Steroids
  Tetracycline
- Chocolate
- Coffee
- Corn, processed
- Cranberry
- Fiber supplements
  (calcium should not
  be taken within

two hours of a fiber
supplement)
- Foods that contain
  oxalic acid
  (spinach, kale,
  rhubarb, or cocoa)
- Fruits, dried
- Heavy exercise
- High-fat diet
- High fiber cereals
  (calcium should not
  be taken within
  two hours after
  eating this)
- High-phosphorus
  foods (white flour
  or soft drinks)
- Honey
- Increased zinc intake
- Whole wheat
- High-protein diet
- Meats and dairy
  products, such as:
  Beef

Butter
Cheese
Chicken
Haddock
Ham
Ice cream
Milk
Turkey
Veal
Yogurt
- Nuts and grains,
  such as:
  Barley
  Bread, white
  Oats
  Peanuts
  Rice
  Soybeans,
    processed
  Walnuts
  Wheat
- Soft drinks
- Sugar
- Tea, black
- Vinegar, white

Finally, while calcium can be beneficial, there are also side effects if you have too much of it in your body.

## ■ Symptoms of Excess Calcium

- ☐ Blocks the absorption of manganese in your body
- ☐ Causes kidney stones
- ☐ Clogs your arteries (predispose you to heart disease)
- ☐ Decreases iron absorption

- ☐ Interferes with the absorption of magnesium
- ☐ Interferes with the absorption of zinc
- ☐ Interferes with the making of vitamin K

# Risk Factors for Osteoporosis

There are many risk factors for osteoporosis. One of the main ones people do not recognize is stress. Adrenal dysfunction is associated with bone loss.

## ■ Other Risk Factors for Osteoporosis

- Alcohol abuse.

- Aluminum-containing antacids. Results of a case-controlled study of over 13,000 people with hip fractures revealed that those taking high doses of PPI antacids (protein pump inhibitors) for more than a year were 2.6 times more likely to break a hip. Those taking modest doses of PPIs regularly for one to four years had an increased risk of hip fracture of 1.2 to 1.6 times those people who did not take PPI antacids.

- Caffeine. Caffeine increases calcium loss. If you drink three cups of coffee a day, for example, you lose 45 mg of calcium. Furthermore, coffee contains twenty-nine different acids which can draw calcium out of your bones. More than 1,000 over-the-counter medications contain caffeine, including weight loss products, cold preparations, pain relievers, and allergy products.

- Certain diseases, such as:
  Anorexia nervosa
  Chronic lower back pain for more than ten years

  Chronic obstructive pulmonary disease (COPD)
  Cushing's disease
  Diabetes
  Fat malabsorption (fats not absorbed well)
  Gallbladder disease
  History of stress fracture
  Hypochlorhydria (not enough acid in the stomach)
  Kidney disease
  Lactose intolerance
  Multiple myeloma
  Nulliparous (having had no children)
  Primary bilary cirrhosis
  Pyercalciuria
  Rheumatoid arthritis
  Scoliosis

- Certain drugs or medications:
  Antidepressants (SSRIs). A study of over 5,000 adults over the age of 50 revealed that SSRIs taken for at least five years was associated with twice the risk of fractures and a reduction of bone density of 4 percent in the hip and 2.4 percent in the spine.

Corticosteroids

*Dilantin* (and other anticonvulsants)

*Heparin*

Isoniazid

Lasix

Lithium

Methotrexate

Tetracycline

- Excessive vitamin A intake.

- Excessive zinc supplementation.

- Fair complexion.

- Family history.*

- Fluoride in drinking water.

- Genetic predisposition.

- High-fat diet.

- Hyperthyroidism (elevated thyroid hormone).

- Lack of exercise.

- Menopause.

- No menstrual cycle for more than six months.

- Nutritional deficiencies:

  Calcium

  Magnesium

  Vitamin D

- Overdose of thyroid medication.

- Overproduction of parathyroid gland.

- Poor diet. Diet high in sulfur amino acids, phosphorus, or chloride (e.g., meat, grains, nuts, dairy products) contribute to the acidic load in the body, which causes increased calcium loss in the urine.

- Small body frame.

- Smoking.

- Sugar intake.

- Surgeries, such as:

  Intestinal bypass surgery for weight control

  Removal of part or all of the intestine

  Total thyroidectomy (thyroid gland is taken out)

- Soft drinks.

*Genome testing is now available from Genova Diagnostics to see if you have this genetic predisposition. (See the Resources on page 183 for more information.)*

Additionally, calcium supplementation can interact with medications. It increases the toxicity of digoxin (a heart medication) and decreases the absorption of ciprofloxacin and most fluroquinolone antibiotics. Calcium can also inhibit the absorption of tetracycline, another antibiotic.

# Acid-Creating Foods

The average American diet includes many foods that, once eaten, create acid in your body. If you eat a majority of acidic foods and not enough alkaline foods, your body has to find alkalizing materials elsewhere to neutralize its pH levels. It often has to resort to using the calcium and protein in your bones. As a result, your bones can become weakened, possibly irrevocably, and your body systems can age at an accelerated pace, resulting in a slew of related problems. The following foods create particularly high acidity levels in your body.

- Chocolate
- Dairy products, such as butter, cheese, ice cream, milk, and yogurt
- Drinks, such as beer, black tea, coffee, and soft drinks
- Fish, such as haddock
- Fruit, such as blueberries, cranberries, and dried fruit
- Grains, such as barley, oats, rice, wheat, and white bread

- Honey
- Meat products, such as beef, chicken, ham, turkey, and veal
- Nuts, such as peanuts and walnuts
- Processed soybeans
- Sugar
- Vegetables, such as corn
- White vinegar

## Magnesium

Magnesium is the fourth most abundant mineral in the body. Fifty percent of the magnesium in your body is found in your bones, which would make it easy to see why magnesium is required to maintain bone health. Magnesium plays many roles in keeping your bones healthy. It increases the absorption of calcium and activates Vitamin D and bone-building osteoblasts. Additionally, magnesium aides in the parathyroid function, which decreases the breakdown of bones. It also increases mineralization density.

In fact, magnesium has over 300 functions in the body. Your calcium-to-magnesium ratio should be about two-to-one.

However, you should be aware that magnesium loss can result from a variety of factors. If you experience any of the items on the following list, be sure to have your doctor measure your magnesium levels so you can monitor them afterwards.

## ■ Causes of Magnesium Deficiency

- Alcoholism
- Antibiotics (gentamicin, carbenicillin, or amphotericin B)
- Asthma medications (beta-agonists or epinephrine)
- Caffeine intake
- Cyclosporine, which prevents organ transplant rejection
- Diarrhea
- Digoxin use (heart medication)
- Diuretics (water pills)
- Drugs used for chemotherapy (cis-platinum, vinblastine, or bleomycin)

- Excessive fiber intake
- Excessive sugar intake
- Extreme athletic competition
- Foods high in oxalic acid (almonds, cocoa, spinach, tea)
- Laxatives
- Phosphates in soft drinks
- Steroids
- Stress
- Surgery
- Trans fatty acids
- Trauma

Like calcium, you can also get magnesium through some magnesium-rich foods.

## ■ Food Sources of Magnesium

- Almonds
- Apricots, dried
- Avocados
- Brazil nuts
- Buckwheat
- Cashews
- Cheddar cheese
- Coconut
- Collard leaves
- Corn
- Dandelion greens

- Dark green vegetables
- Dates
- Figs, dried
- Kelp
- Parsley
- Peanuts
- Prunes, dried
- Pumpkin seeds
- Rice, brown
- Rye

- Sesame seeds
- Shrimp
- Soybeans
- Spinach, raw
- Sunflower seeds
- Swiss chard
- Tofu
- Wheat bran
- Wheat germ
- Wheat grain
- Yeast, brewer's

## Boron

Boron is a trace mineral, which means the body only requires it in a small amount. It is needed for calcium metabolism and also helps activate vitamin D and estrogen. Boron, along with vitamin D, increases the mineral content in your bone and also increases cartilage formation and helps maintain memory.

### ■ Food Sources of Boron

- Almonds
- Apples
- Broccoli
- Cauliflower
- Dates
- Grapes
- Green leafy vegetables, such as kale
- Hazelnuts
- Honey
- Legumes
- Peaches
- Peanuts
- Pears
- Prunes
- Raisins
- Tomatoes

## Zinc

Zinc is needed for the formation of bone and it enhances the biochemical actions of Vitamin D in the body. It is very important for your overall physical and mental health. Over one hundred enzymes in the body need zinc as a cofactor, or a molecule to which another molecule must bind in order to activate it.

### ■ Symptoms of Zinc Deficiency

- ☐ Acne
- ☐ Anemia
- ☐ Anorexia
- ☐ Arthritis
- ☐ Behavioral disturbances
- ☐ Brittle nails
- ☐ Craving for sugary foods
- ☐ Dandruff
- ☐ Decreased ability to taste
- ☐ Decreased desire for protein-rich foods
- ☐ Decreased sense of smell
- ☐ Decreased sexual function
- ☐ Delayed sexual maturation
- ☐ Diarrhea
- ☐ Eczema
- ☐ Enlargement of the spleen and liver
- ☐ Fatigue
- ☐ Frontal headaches
- ☐ Growth retardation
- ☐ Hair loss

☐ Immune deficiencies

☐ Impaired nerve conduction

☐ Impaired wound healing

☐ Impotence

☐ Infertility

☐ Low sperm count

☐ Memory impairment

☐ Negative nitrogen balance

☐ Nerve damage

☐ Night blindness

☐ Poor appetite

☐ Psoriasis

☐ Reduced salivation

☐ Sleep disturbances

☐ Stretch marks

☐ White spots on nails

## ■ Factors that Can Predispose You to a Zinc Deficiency

- Aging (zinc absorption decreases with age)
- AIDS
- Alcoholism
- Anorexia nervosa
- Caffeinated beverages
- Calcium supplementation
- Celiac disease
- Certain medications, such as:
  *Cortisone*
  Some diuretics (water pills)
  Tetracycline
- Chronic renal (kidney) failure
- Cirrhosis
- Cystic fibrosis
- Excess copper
- Foods rich in phytic acid, such as unleavened bread, raw beans, seeds, nuts, and grains
- Hemolytic anemia
- Infection
- Inflammatory bowel disease
- Iron supplementation
- Nephritic syndrome
- Pancreatic insufficiency
- Pancreatitis
- Rheumatoid arthritis
- Short bowel syndrome
- Smoking
- Surgery
- Teas containing tannin

## ■ Food Sources of Zinc

- Almonds
- Beef
- Black pepper
- Brazil nuts
- Buckwheat
- Chicken
- Chili powder
- Cinnamon
- Egg yolk
- Ginger root
- Ground round steak

- Hazelnuts
- Lamb chops
- Lima beans
- Milk, dry; nonfat
- Mustard
- Oats

- Oysters, fresh
- Paprika
- Peanuts
- Pecans
- Rye
- Sardines

- Soy lecithin
- Split peas
- Thyme
- Walnuts
- Whole wheat

## Copper

Copper plays an important role in bone metabolism and turnover. Copper is involved with the differentiation and proliferation of mesenchymal stem cells that develop osteoblasts in the body. Osteoblasts make bone. Copper and zinc have to sit in appropriate ratios in the body. Usually 10 to 15 mgs of zinc to 1 mg of copper are needed.

### ■ Food Sources of Copper

- Almonds
- Barley
- Beef liver
- Brazil nuts
- Buckwheat
- Butter
- Carrots
- Clams

- Coconut
- Cod liver oil
- Garlic
- Hazelnuts
- Lamb chops
- Olive oil
- Oysters
- Peanuts

- Pecans
- Pork loin
- Rye grain
- Shrimp
- Split peas, dry
- Sunflower oil
- Walnuts

## Manganese

Manganese is needed for the repair of soft bone and connective tissue and is used for bone growth and maintainence. Too much calcium can decrease the absorption of manganese. It is also required for the production of estrogen and progesterone. Manganese also aids in protein digestion and syntheses, is essential for a healthy nervous system, and is needed for the utilization of vitamins B and C in adrenal health.

Levels of manganese that are too low can have negative consequences as well. Your hair and nails will not grow as well if you are deficient in manganese. Additionally, low levels of manganese are associated with low HDL (good cholesterol), impaired carbohydrate and lipid metabolism, decreased fatty acid production, impaired coordination, loss of hair color, and skin rashes. Phytates (the main storage form of phosphorus), which are in bread and aluminum, can also decrease manganese levels.

### ■ Food Sources of Manganese

- Avocados
- Bay leaves
- Brazil nuts
- Buckwheat
- Cloves
- Ginger
- Hazelnuts
- Oatmeal
- Pecans
- Seaweed
- Tea
- Thyme
- Whole wheat

### Silicon

Silicon is a trace mineral that has been shown to increase bone mineral density. It is found in many forms, but the only form that is useful to humans is orthosilicic acid. Foods that are high in fiber usually contain silicon. The recommended dose is 1 to 5 mg a day. High dosages can cause kidney stone production.

### ■ Food Sources of Silicon

- Apples
- Celery
- Cherries
- Endive
- Legumes
- Oats
- Onions
- Oranges
- Rice bran
- Root vegetables
- Unrefined grains

### Phosphorus

Phosphorus regulates bone formation, inhibits bone re-absorption, and affects the regulation of calcium. Most Americans eat enough phosphorus-containing foods that low phosphorus levels are rarely seen.

### ■ Food Sources of Phosphorus

- Almonds
- Beef liver
- Brazil nuts
- Brewer's yeast
- Brown rice
- Cashews
- Cheddar cheese
- Chicken
- Dried pinto beans

- Dried soy beans
- Eggs
- English walnuts
- Garlic
- Hulked sesame seeds
- Kelp

- Millet
- Peanuts
- Pearled barley
- Pecans
- Pumpkin seeds
- Rye grain

- Scallops
- Squash seeds
- Sunflower seeds
- Wheat
- Wheat bran
- Wheat germ

## Vitamins $B_6$, $B_{12}$, and Folate

Low levels of vitamins $B_6$, $B_{12}$, and folate are common in people with osteoporosis. High levels of homocysteine (see section on heart disease) are also a risk factor for osteoporosis. High homocysteine levels interfere with collagen cross-linking, leading to a bone matrix that is defective and not as strong. This may be due to the fact that high amounts of homocysteine are associated with vitamin $B_{12}$ deficiency. Studies have shown that low levels of vitamin $B_{12}$ are associated with low bone mineral density in the hip.

## Vitamin D

Vitamin D is needed for the absorption of calcium and the mineralization of bone. The recommended daily amount you need is determined by measuring your blood levels of vitamin D.

Vitamin D also has neurotransmitter and neurological function. There are vitamin D receptors in your bones, intestines, brain, breasts, and lymphocytes. Vitamin D furthermore affects the immune system by having anti-inflammatory effects, and it also modulates transcription of several of your genes.

Suboptimal levels of vitamin D are associated with other diseases besides bone loss.

## ■ Diseases Associated With Suboptimal Vitamin D Levels

- Ankylosing spondylitis
- Back pain
- Breast cancer
- Colon cancer
- Depression
- Diabetes

- Epilepsy
- Grave's disease
- Heart disease
- Hypertension (high blood pressure)
- Lupus
- Migraine headaches

- Multiple sclerosis (MS)
- Osteoarthritis
- Parkinson's disease
- PCOS
- Rheumatiod arthritis

Vitamin D is mainly available through sunlight. You make it in your skin from exposure to the sun. Topical sunscreens block vitamin D production by 97 to 100 percent. Dairy products, fish and fish liver oils, liver, sweet potatoes, and dandelion greens also contain some vitamin D. Supplementation with vitamin D is best done with vitamin $D_3$. New studies have shown that you may need more vitamin D than healthcare providers previously thought. Therefore, it is very important to have your vitamin D levels measured regularly.

## Vitamin K

Vitamin K helps your body maintain a hormone called osteocalcin, which is needed for bone mineralization. There are two types of natural vitamin K: $K_1$ and $K_2$. $K_2$ is the type of vitamin K that is responsible for bone mineralization. However, $K_1$ can also help with bone formation because it is converted to $K_2$ in the body.

Vitamin K supplementation has been shown to help prevent and treat osteoporosis, specifically vitamin $K_2$.

$K_1$ is called phylloquinone and is found in leafy green vegetables and soybean oil.

$K_2$ is called menaquinone and is made in your intestinal tract by friendly bacteria. Of the vitamin K your body uses, 75 percent is $K_2$. Studies have shown that those who intake higher vitamin $K_2$ levels have a reduction in mortality from coronary heart disease and overall mortality.

Both $K_1$ and $K_2$ are fat soluble. However, unlike other fat-soluble vitamins, vitamin K is not stored in the body.

Vitamin K has also been shown to decrease vascular calcification, which are calcium plaques in the arteries that supply blood to the heart. A study has found that low levels of vitamin K impair activation of osteocalcin (the chief bone matrix protein) and consequently, less bone is formed.

## ■ Causes of Vitamin K Deficiency

- Antibiotic use
- Cholesterol-lowering drugs
- Decreased intake of green, leafy vegetables
- Excess vitamin A
- Excess vitamin E
- Gallstones
- Liver disease
- Synthetic estrogen use
- Unhealthy intestinal tract

Furthermore, consumption of hydrogenated and partially-hydrogenated fats (trans fatty acids) produces hydrogenated vitamin K. This type is not well absorbed and has been shown to not aid in bone production.

Twenty-five percent of the vitamin K that you use comes from your diet. Studies have shown that vitamin K intake on a daily basis must be at least 100 micrograms to maintain optimal bone health.

### ■ Food Sources of Vitamin K

- Asparagus
- Beef
- Broccoli
- Cheese
- Egg yolks
- Green beans
- Green cabbage

- Ham
- Lettuce
- Liver (beef, pork, chicken)
- Oats
- Peaches
- Potatoes

- Raisins
- Spinach
- Tomatoes
- Turnip greens
- Watercress
- Whole wheat

If you are on an anticoagulant such as *Coumadin*, consult your doctor as to how much vitamin K-rich foods or supplementation you may need. Studies have revealed that bone density is reduced in some patients who take *Coumadin*. Likewise, an increased risk of bone fracture has been associated with long-term use of *Coumadin*. Research has shown that taking *Coumadin* with a low dose of vitamin K (100 micrograms a day) can be beneficial and safe. Still, you should consult your healthcare practitioner before beginning vitamin K supplementation if you are taking *Coumadin*.

A recent study also revealed that supplementation of vitamin $K_2$ improves the effectiveness of bisphosphonates, which are medications used to treat osteoporosis.

### Strontium

Strontium is an element that is naturally found in your bones. It is currently being researched as a treatment for osteoporosis. Strontium promotes bone formation and decreases bone resorption. Studies have found a 37 percent reduction in vertebral fractures and a 40 percent reduction in non-vertebral fractures when people were supplementing with strontium.

A study published in the *New England Journal of Medicine* in 2004 suggests that strontium may be as good a treatment for bone loss as other medications, like *Fosamax* (alendronate), *Actonel* (risedronate), *Evista* (raloxifene), and *Forteo* (teriparatide), which is an injectable hormone. Another study published the next year produced similar results.

## Amino Acids

Amino acids are the building blocks for proteins. They also contribute to bone structure. Studies have shown that the amino acids L-arginine and L-lysine stimulate osteoblast (bone growth) activity. Amino acid levels can be measured in your body by doing a blood test or a twenty-four-hour urine test for amino acids.

## Bioflavones

Bioflavones such as rutin, quercetin, and hesperidin have been shown to stimulate bone morphogenetic proteins, which increase bone formation. Bioflavones are contained in foods such as onions, peppers, garlic, black currants, blueberries, red berries, green tea, and buckwheat. A particular kind of bioflavone called "ipriflavone" is a synthetic bioflavone. Studies have shown that 200 mg of ipriflavone three times a day increases bone density by 2 to 6 percent after one year of use. Side effects include lymphocytopenia (low lymphocyte count). Therefore, ipriflavone should be used only under the direction of a healthcare practitioner.

| SUPPLEMENTATION TO TREAT OSTEOPOROSIS | | |
|---|---|---|
| Supplements | Dosage | Considerations |
| Boron | 1 to 5 mg once a day | |
| Calcium | 500 to 1,200 mg daily, in dosages no larger than 500 mg | Use calcium hydroxyapatite or calcium citrate. Do not use calcium carbonate. Although there are people deficient in calcium, there is a danger in taking too much calcium. Do not ingest more than 1,000 to 1,200 mg of calcium a day. |
| Copper | 1 to 2 mg once a day | Your copper-to-zinc ratio is very important for your health. Also, do not take copper supplement cupric oxide, which has a very low bioavailability. |
| EPA/DHA (fish oil) | 500 to 1,000 mg once a day | Choose a source that contains vitamin E to prevent oxidation. |

| | | |
|---|---|---|
| Gamma-linolenic acid (GLA) | 240 mg once a day | It is important to maintain the proper ratio of omega-6 fatty acids to omega-3 fatty acids. |
| Ipriflavone | 150 to 200 mg three times a day | |
| Magnesium | 400 to 800 mg once a day | Consult healthcare provider for dosage if you have kidney disease. Discontinue use and see your doctor if you experience abdominal pain. Take a lower dose if it causes diarrhea. |
| Manganese | 5 to 10 mg once a day | Do not take high dosages if you are prone to kidney stones or gout. |
| Vitamin $B_9$ (folic acid) | 500 mcg once a day | High doses can deplete your body of other vitamins in the B complex. |
| Vitamin $B_{12}$ (cobalamin) | 1,000 mcg twice a day | High doses can deplete your body of other vitamins in the B complex. |
| Vitamin D | Varies (see doctor for dosage) | Have your blood levels measured by your healthcare provider, who will then determine proper dosage. |
| Vitamin K | 150 mcg once a day | High dosages can cause toxicity. Consult your healthcare provider before taking if you are on an anticoagulant. $K_2$ is particularly effective at maintaining bone structure. |
| Zinc | 25 mg once a day | The best supplements are zinc picolinate and zinc citrate. If you are taking zinc and iron supplements, take one in the morning and one in the evening. (Taking them together reduces the efficiency of both.) |

Nutrients alone are not enough to prevent osteoporosis. Approximately 93 percent of women who do not take hormones will have a bone fracture by the age of eighty-five. Estrogen helps maintain bone and therefore retards the progression of osteoporosis. It controls the absorption of calcium into the bone and stimulates the production of calcitonin, which is a hormone that protects bone. Additionally, other hormones work with estrogen to protect the bones. Progesterone and testosterone build bone, but testosterone also makes the bone strong. Even the hormone melatonin helps prevent bone loss by signaling the production of bone matrix proteins and increasing the production of growth hormone. Melatonin also inhibits osteoclast formation. Osteoclasts break down bone in the body.

Furthermore, melatonin promotes osteoblast proteins and procollagen type-1 c-peptide, both of which aid in bone building.

Researchers are now looking at bone turnover (breakdown) as a better indicator of fracture risk from osteoporosis than bone density. Measuring the biochemical markers of bone turnover, called urinary N-telopeptides, are a good way to accurately gauge response to hormone replacement therapy or drug treatment to see if they are helping your bone health. N-telopeptides are a product of the breakdown of a kind of collagen found in your bones. When bones break down, these peptides are excreted in your urine. Therefore, N-telopeptides are specific markers of bone breakdown. Testing of urinary telopeptides is a very effective way of measuring these levels. By doing this, your doctor can fully evaluate the status of your bones and the rate at which they are breaking down or forming. Contact Genova Diagnostic Laboratory (see page 183) for availability of this test. Urine levels of telopeptides usually decrease within thirty days of starting hormonal therapy. It is a good idea to have this test done one to three months after beginning treatment for bone loss, no matter how young or old you are.

Some women inherit a gene that decreases the absorption of calcium in their bones. Therefore, your family history plays a role in your personal risk of osteoporosis. Genome testing is now available to see if you have this genetic predisposition by Genova Diagnostic Laboratory under their *Genovations* testing. (See the Resources section on page 183.)

## OVARIAN CANCER

*See* Cancer.

## PAINFUL INTERCOURSE

*See* Endometriosis.

## PAINFUL MENSTRUAL CYCLES

*See* Endometriosis.

## PELVIC PAIN

*See* Endometriosis.

# PERIMENOPAUSE

*See* Menopause.

# POLYCYSTIC OVARIAN SYNDROME (PCOS)

Polycystic ovarian syndrome (PCOS) is yet another female issue that results from an imbalance of hormones. It is characterized by irregular menstrual cycles and excess testosterone production. Women who have PCOS may have difficulties getting pregnant. PCOS can also cause changes in appearance, and if untreated it can lead to serious health issues, such as diabetes or heart disease.

Many scientists believe that PCOS has a hereditary component. Your chance of developing PCOS is higher if other women in your family have PCOS, irregular periods, or diabetes. You can inherit PCOS from your mother's or your father's side of the family.

PCOS is a risk factor for other major ailments, including obesity and insulin resistance, which can lead to diabetes. Studies have shown that women with PCOS store more fat and burn calories at a slower rate than women who do not have PCOS.

## ◼ Signs and Symptoms of PCOS

PCOS affects as many as one in fifteen women. Symptoms usually begin in the teen years, and can include:

- ☐ Abnormal lipid profile
- ☐ Acne
- ☐ Alopecia (hair loss on the head)
- ☐ Cysts on the ovaries
- ☐ Decreased levels of sex hormone binding globulin (SHBG)
- ☐ Depression
- ☐ Elevated insulin levels/insulin resistance
- ☐ Elevated lutenizing hormone (LH)
- ☐ High blood pressure
- ☐ High testosterone levels
- ☐ Hirsutism (excessive body hair)
- ☐ Infertility
- ☐ Irregular or absent menstrual cycles
- ☐ Obesity
- ☐ Oily skin
- ☐ Recurrent miscarriages
- ☐ Skin tags

## DIAGNOSING PCOS

There is not one surefire way to diagnose PCOS. That is why, if you are experiencing any of the symptoms associated with the disease, it is important to see a doctor to get a proper diagnosis. The doctor will ask questions about your general health, symptoms, and menstrual cycles. He or she will complete a physical exam to check for signs of PCOS, such as high blood pressure or extra body hair. The doctor will also check your body mass index (BMI) to determine if you are at an appropriate weight. Finally, he or she will conduct various lab tests, including salivary testing, to check blood sugar, insulin, and other hormone levels. This will help rule out other hormonal problems that may have similar symptoms.

Your doctor should be able to diagnose PCOS without having to do a pelvic ultrasound, but sometimes he or she will conduct one anyway to check for cysts on the ovaries or to rule out other problems.

### ■ Causes of PCOS

- Follistatin. Studies have shown that the high levels of testosterone and insulin in patients with PCOS are linked. This link is a gene called follistatin. In the body, follistatin has two functions. It plays a role in the development of the ovaries and it is also needed to make insulin.

- High LH/FSH ratio. In a woman who has PCOS, the luteinizing hormone (LH)/follicle-stimulating hormone (FSH) ratio is, a majority of the time, abnormally high.

- Stress. Stress can also be a contributing factor to the development of PCOS. Recent studies have shown that many women with PCOS cannot process cortisol effectively, which can lead to elevated cortisol levels. This, in turn, can result in more stress. Likewise, women who are under a lot of stress make too much prolactin. This may affect the ovaries' ability to produce hormones in a balanced manner.

### ■ Treating PCOS

Once diagnosed, it is important to start treatment for PCOS. Treatment for the disease varies, and may include:

- Antioxidants

- Certain medications, such as:

    Birth control pills, which regulate menstrual cycles and help reduce facial hair and acne

    Diabetes medications, which help control insulin and blood sugar levels

    Fertility medicines, which can help women who are having difficulty getting pregnant

- Exercise

- Fiber

- Healthy eating

- Increasing intake of essential fatty acids, such as fish oil

- Low glycemic index diet

- Menstrual-regulating drugs, such as oral contraceptives or natural progesterone

- Stress reduction

- Weight control

Walking is a great exercise that many people can do. For most people, it isn't too strenuous. It can lower the risk factors for PCOS and associated diseases, and can also help you lose weight.

Most women who suffer from PCOS can benefit from losing weight. Losing as little as ten pounds can help straighten out hormonal imbalances.

Eating heart-healthy can also help when treating PCOS. A diet with lots of vegetables, fruits, beans, nuts, and whole grains is beneficial. Lentils, chickpeas, and broccoli specifically will also help decrease insulin levels.

As is with other diseases, smoking does not help. However, this stands especially true for PCOS since untreated PCOS can lead to heart disease, which is only made worse by smoking. Additionally, smoking can lead to higher androgen levels, which can worsen PCOS symptoms. Quitting would be beneficial in treating PCOS.

| SUPPLEMENTATION TO TREAT PCOS BY LOWERING BLOOD SUGAR | | |
|---|---|---|
| **Supplements** | **Dosage** | **Considerations** |
| Alpha lipoic acid | 200 to 600 mg | |
| B-vitamin complex | 50 to100 mg | |
| Biotin | 4 to 8 mg | |
| Chromium picolinate | 600 to 1,200 micrograms | |
| CLA | 1,000 to 3,000 mg | |
| Coenzyme Q-10 | 30 to 300 mg | |
| Inositol | Varies (see doctor for dosage) | |
| Magnesium | 400 to 800 mg | |
| Manganese | 5 to10 mg | |
| Taurine | 1,000 to 3,000 mg | Taurine levels are low when you are stressed |
| Vanadium | 20 to 50 mg | |
| Vitamin C | 1,000 to 3,000 mg | |
| Vitamin D | Varies (see doctor for dosage) | |
| Zinc | 25 to 50 mg | |

Additionally, supplementation with the herbs fenugreek, gymnema sylvestre, cinnamon, black cohosh, and chasteberry can be beneficial.

High doses of niacin, a B-vitamin that occurs naturally in plants and animals, should be avoided in people with PCOS since it can worsen insulin sensitivity.

# POSTPARTUM DEPRESSION

After a pregnancy, your body resets its hormonal levels, which sometimes results in an imbalance in hormonal function. Because of this, some women experience postpartum depression. (It is estimated that about 10 percent of new moms experience this.)

When you deliver, the drop in estrogen is two thousand times greater than the drop in estrogen you experience just before your cycle begins. Progesterone levels also fall abruptly at delivery, which can trigger depression as well. (This also occurs if a woman has a C-section.) Taking natural hormones postpartum may be necessary to help rebalance your hormonal levels.

After delivery, thyroid hormone levels can also be dysfunctional. In fact, postpartum thyroid disorders occur in 5 to 10 percent of women. It is important to measure hormonal levels since some of the symptoms of low thyroid function (hypothyroidism) are very similar to the symptoms of estrogen and/or progesterone loss. Furthermore, postpartum thyroid dysfunction can occur up to three years after delivery.

There is no way to pinpoint the cause of postpartum depression. Physical, emotional, and lifestyle factors can all contribute. Likewise, it is difficult to diagnose postpartum depression. To tell the difference between the baby blues (a short-term, lesser degree of depression) and postpartum depression, your doctor will likely administer a depression-screening questionnaire and a few blood tests, including thyroid studies.

---

# Risk Factors for Postpartum Depression

Postpartum depression is not exclusive to first-time moms. It can occur after the birth of any child. A new mom's risk of developing postpartum depression increases if the mom:

- Did not want or expect the pregnancy

- Experienced a great deal of stress during the year before delivery

- Experienced a marital conflict

- Had postpartum depression after a previous pregnancy

- Has a history of depression

- Has a weak support system from family and friends

---

## ■ Symptoms of Postpartum Depression

Postpartum depression symptoms last longer and are more severe than symptoms of the baby blues. Mothers suffering from postpartum depression may experience:

- ☐ Decreased appetite
- ☐ Difficulty bonding with the baby
- ☐ Fatigue, overwhelming at times
- ☐ Feeling shameful or guilty without cause
- ☐ Increased irritability and anger
- ☐ Insomnia
- ☐ Loss of sexual interest
- ☐ Mood swings, severe at times
- ☐ Social withdrawal
- ☐ Thoughts of harming themselves or their babies

# Preconception Medicine:
# Things to Consider Before You Conceive

The health of the mother is a very important part of whether her child will be healthy or not. Therefore, if you are planning on conceiving, it would be beneficial to have a preconception medicine evaluation done to see what all your hormone levels are.

Preconception medicine is a field of medicine that metabolic and anti-aging physicians specialize in. These doctors look at the health of the mother before she conceives. Studies have shown that if the mother is taking omega-3-fatty acids—like fish oil—when she gets pregnant and continues to take them throughout the pregnancy, her baby will have a higher IQ, a smaller chance of developing ADD/ADHD, and a lower rate of dyslexia.

An evaluation for Preconception Medicine by a Metabolic/Anti-Aging specialist would include a salivary test for your female and adrenal hormones, thyroid studies, basic blood work (like your cholesterol and blood sugar), lab studies to determine if you have any nutritional deficiencies (vitamins, minerals, fatty acids, organic acids, and amino acids are all checked), and studies to determine if your liver and gastrointestinal tract are working optimally, along with a test of the toxins in your body, such as toxic metals, phthalates (compounds used in the production of plastics), volatile solvents, PCBs, and pesticides.

Are your female hormones balanced? Are you nutritionally sound? Is your thyroid working optimally? Are you stressed? These are some of the questions that affect the health of your baby and whether you will be able to conceive. Preconception testing checks all these factors out.

## Infertility/Difficulty Conceiving

There are many other overlooked factors that are related to infertility and difficulty conceiving. Alcohol abuse, cigarette smoking, and recreational drugs all affect your health and, subsequently, the health of your child.

● *Alcohol abuse.* Women do not metabolize alcohol as quickly as men do, so when women drink, the alcohol stays in their systems much longer than it would stay in a man's system. Women who abuse alcohol have a higher rate of premature births, delivering children with birth defects, and still-births. However, women don't have to abuse alcohol to learn its effects on their fertility. Regular alcohol use can cause an increase in miscarriages. Alcohol abuse also leads to declines in estrogen and testosterone at an earlier age, which can decrease fertility.

Alcohol use also affects the menstrual cycle. Studies have shown that women who drink alcohol have more severe PMS than those who do not drink. Additionally, these women have more menstrual cycles that do not include ovulation. Furthermore, women who drink alcohol on a regular basis have cycles that are more variable in length.

Many studies now link continual use of alcohol to an increase in breast cancer risk.

- *Cigarette smoking.* Cigarette smoking affects the balance of your hormones. Women who smoke have higher rates of ovarian cysts and a higher risk of endometriosis. Cigarette smoking can also lead to premature ovarian failure (POF). Cigarette smoke is toxic to the follicles in your ovaries. There are numerous studies that show infertility is associated with cigarette smoking. One study showed that women who smoke are 57 to 75 percent less likely to get pregnant than women who don't smoke. Of the smokers who were able to get pregnant, it took longer for them to conceive. Additionally, women who have in vitro fertilization have lower success rates if they smoke.

Smokers are also more likely to give birth to lower birth weight or premature children. Their children are also are more likely to have fetal growth retardation, which is when the baby's weight is below the tenth percentile for its gestational age. Daughters born to mothers who smoked during pregnancy may grow up to have fertility issues of their own. This may be because smoking kills some of the primordial follicles in the developing daughter.

Smoking can also lead to early menopause—this includes secondhand smoke. When you smoke, the nicotine may result in your body not making as much estrogen as it should. Nicotine also affects your mood and sleep regulation. If your estrogen level is low and you smoke, the pH of your stomach and intestines are affected. When this happens, your body is not able to absorb calcium, magnesium, B vitamins, and other nutrients. Additionally, if the pH of your stomach is changed, you may also have symptoms of reflux, such as heartburn. Cigarette smoking also significantly increases your risk of developing breast cancer.

● *Recreational drug use.* Recreational drug use also affects your baby and your fertility. Women who smoke marijuana have changes in ovulation that affect their ability to become pregnant. Marijuana use also causes more frequent miscarriages. Women who smoke marijuana when they are pregnant can have children with abnormal brain function, small head circumference, reduced height, and lower birth weight. (Keep in mind, it is not just women. When men smoke, marijuana affects sperm development and lowers testosterone, both of which can affect a woman's ability to conceive.)

Marijuana disrupts brain functions that regulate hormone production. Luteinizing hormone (LH), which is the hormone that triggers ovulation during your cycle, is lowered when you smoke marijuana. If you don't ovulate, you cannot get pregnant.

The chemicals in marijuana, such as THC, also compete with estradiol (E2) for binding at the receptor sites. If this happens, the sites are not available for estrogen to bind and women can have some of the symptoms of estrogen loss, including a decrease in fertility. Marijuana can also increase prolactin, the hormone that is high when you breastfeed. High prolactin levels decrease production of your sex hormones that are involved in producing a normal menstrual cycle.

Of course, marijuana is not the only recreational drug that can affect fertility. Cocaine use changes how your fallopian tubes function and may interfere with your ability to get pregnant. Cocaine and ecstasy may disrupt your cycle and cause irregularity, which also affects fertility.

## Additional Complications

There are some additional factors that can affect your pregnancy and your children that have not been previously discussed. Diet, certain herbs, and stress can all have negative effects on pregnancy and childbirth.

● *Diet.* Your diet can also affect your ability to get pregnant and how healthy your child may be. Low-fat diets are to be avoided. If your body's fat content falls below 20 to 22 percent, it can influence your ability to have a baby. Being severely overweight also affects pregnancy rates.

High-soy diets should also be avoided, because they may interfere with the body's ability to make estrogen and progesterone. Too much soy can also interfere with estrogen and progesterone's abilities to bind to their receptor sites.

- *Herbs.* There are some herbs that have been found to have a negative effect on fertility and pregnancy. They include:

| | | |
|---|---|---|
| Black cohosh | Ephedra | Passionflower |
| Blue cohosh | Evening primrose | Red clover |
| Cat's claw | Feverfew | St. John's wort |
| Chaste tree | Ginseng | Wild yam |
| Dong quai | Gotu kola | |

Men should be wary as well. Herbs can affect sperm count and viability, so men should check with their doctors if they consume any of the herbs on the list.

- *Stress.* Stress can lower estradiol, testosterone, progesterone, and DHEA production. Studies have shown that if a mother suffers prenatal stress, her children have an increased risk of developing ADD, learning disorders, increased anxiety, impaired coping skills, depression, and abnormal social behavior.

A mother's elevated stress hormones can cause changes in the brain of her offspring, due to the disturbances that may occur in the hypothalamic-pituitary-adrenal pathways. The hypothalamus and pituitary are where the stimulating hormones are made that affect the ovaries and the adrenal glands. A child born under these circumstances may have less cortisol receptors in his or her brain, high cortisol production in response to stress, changes in the feedback mechanism involving corticotrophin-releasing hormone (CRH), and decreased GABA (calming neurotransmitter) effectiveness. Furthermore, endorphin, the "feel good" chemical messenger system, may be negatively affected in the child if the mother is stressed. Additionally, children born to mothers who suffered prenatal stress may have delayed puberty due to alterations in follicle-stimulating hormone (FSH) and LH, the hormones produced in the brain that regulate ovarian production (in boys, this would affect testicular production).

## ◼ Treating Postpartum Depression

- Antidepressants. Antidepressants are a proven treatment for postpartum depression. It's important to discuss this method of treatment with your doctor before beginning, especially if you are breast-feeding, since medications can enter your baby's body through your breast milk.

- Counseling. Talking it out with a mental help professional can help you cope with your feelings, set goals, and solve problems.

- Estrogen and/or progesterone replacement. This can help counteract the rapid decline in estrogen and progesterone that occurs after childbirth. This can help ease the signs and symptoms of postpartum depression.

- Therapy. Family or marital therapy can sometimes help. As with counseling, talking it out with family and a mental health professional can be extremely therapeutic.

With appropriate treatment, symptoms usually improve and alleviate after a few months, but have been known to last up to a year in some cases.

### SUPPLEMENTATION TO TREAT POSTPARTUM DEPRESSION

| Supplements | Dosage | Considerations |
| --- | --- | --- |
| Omega-3 fatty acids (fish oil) | 1,000 to 2,000 mg once a day | Be sure to take pharmaceutical-grade fish oil that is guaranteed to be free of mercury |

## PREMATURE OVARIAN DECLINE (POD)

Premature ovarian decline (POD) and premature ovarian failure (POF) are similar ailments. With POD, hormone production begins to decrease at an early age. However, women with POD still have follicles in their ovaries and still experience menstrual cycles. POF refers to a loss of normal hormonal function at an early age.

Premature ovarian decline (POD) is the term used to describe the early phase of a decrease in ovarian hormone production. This term was coined by Dr. Elizabeth Vliet in her book *It's My Ovaries, Stupid.*

Some women will experience a decline in hormonal function long before perimenopause. There may be a decline in estrogen, progesterone, or testosterone. For some time, physicians and scientists have described estrogen dominance as excess amounts of estrogen that do not balance with progesterone. Studies show that some women can have low estrogen or testosterone levels even though their progesterone and FSH (follicle stimulating hormone) levels are normal and the woman is still menstruating.

# Risk Factors for POD

- Body weight—thinner women have earlier onset
- Decline in estradiol (E2)
- Living at high altitudes
- Malnutrition
- Mother had an early onset of menopause
- Never having been pregnant
- Vegetarian diet

## ■ Causes of POD (as described by Dr. Vliet in her book *It's My Ovaries Stupid*)

- Chronic dieting

- Cigarette smoking, which damages ovarian follicles

- Compulsive exercise

- Discontinuing birth control pills after long-term usage (especially high-progestin pills)

- Eating disorders, such as anorexia or bulimia, that suppress the hypothalamus and its regulation of the ovaries

- Hypothalmic dysfunction due to high intake of soy or other excitotoxins (glutamate, MSG, or aspartame)

- Hysterectomy without ovarian removal

- PCOS

- Postpartum (the time after delivery)

- Thyroid disorders

- Toxic exposures, such as black widow spider bites, Lyme disease, or pesticides

- Tubal ligation, commonly known as "getting your tubes tied," as a method of birth control

- Viral oophoritis (viral infection that damages the ovary)

Premature ovarian failure (POF) is not entirely the same as POD. POF is defined as the end of menstrual cycles before the age of thirty-five while follicle-stimulating hormone (FSH) levels are elevated (above 20 mIU/mL). FSH is the hormone that regulates the development, growth, pubertal maturation, and reproductive process in the human body.

## ■ Symptoms of POF

Many of the symptoms of POF are similar to symptoms of menopause.

☐ Decreased sexual desire            ☐ Irritability

☐ Difficulty concentrating           ☐ Night sweats

☐ Hot flashes                        ☐ Shorter life span

☐ Irregular menstrual cycles         ☐ Vaginal dryness

## ■ Causes of POF

POF can develop when there are few or no responsive follicles left in the ovaries. ("Responsive" follicles are the follicles that release estrogen while maturing and eventually release an egg. When there are few or none left, it is called follicle depletion.) It can also result from follicles that don't respond properly (follicle dysfunction). However, more often than not there is no definitive cause of POF.

• Follicle depletion. Follicle depletion can be caused by chromosomal defects or by exposure to toxins.

• Follicle dysfunction. Follicle dysfunction usually arises from autoimmune diseases. A woman's body sometimes produces antibodies against her own ovarian tissue, which can harm the follicles that contain eggs.

---

# Risk Factors for POF

There are many reasons why women may experience POF, such as early loss of follicles in the ovaries, viruses, endocrine disruptors, autoimmune diseases, or any other disorder that prevents the ovaries from functioning normally. However, there are only two main risk factors for POF:

• Age. The older you get, the higher your risk of developing POF will be. At age thirty-five, the average woman's risk of developing POF is one in 250.

• Family history. If POF runs in your family, your risk of developing the disease is greater.

However, in her book *It's My Ovaries, Stupid,* Dr. Elizabeth Vliet looks at many other possible reasons why the ovaries stop functioning at an early age.

## ■ Additional Causes of POF

- Autoimmune disease
- Cessation of birth control pills after long-term use
- Chemotherapy
- Chronic dieting and eating disorders (anorexia, bulimia)
- Cigarette smoking
- Compulsive exercise
- Damage before you were born (in utero) from smoking, alcohol, pesticides, and other chemical exposures
- Genetic abnormalities
- High intake of excitatory amino acids (glutamate, MSG, aspartame)
- High intake of soy
- Hysterectomy without removal of ovaries
- Living at high altitudes
- Malnutrition
- Medications that disrupt the hypothalamic-pituitary-ovarian pathways (antidepressants, antipsychotics, and anticonvulsants)
- Never having been pregnant (more pregnancies lead to later menopause)
- PCOS
- Postpartum (may happen to women who are older when they deliver)
- Radiation exposure
- Recreational drug use (marijuana, cocaine, ecstasy)
- Thin body structure (thinner women have earlier onset)
- Thyroid disorders
- Toxic exposures (black widow spider bites, Lyme disease, pesticides)
- Tubal ligation

- Vegetarian diet

- Viral oophoritis (viral infiltration of the ovary)

## ▇ Treating POF

- Addressing infertility. Infertility is a common complication of POF, and unfortunately, there is no treatment to restore fertility to women who have POF. However, one thing that can be viewed as a type of treatment for infertility is to look into alternate forms of childbirth, such as in vitro fertilization with donor eggs.

- Estrogen therapy. Replacing estrogen can help relieve vaginal dryness and hot flashes. However, if your doctor prescribes estrogen for you, he

---

### DIAGNOSING POF

If you go without a period for three or more months, it's time to see a doctor.

To diagnose POF, doctors will likely ask questions about your symptoms, menstrual patterns, and history of exposure to toxins. Most sufferers show few symptoms, so a physical exam (including a pelvic exam) is usually necessary as well.

The physical exam contains a few blood tests:

- FSH test. Women with POF usually have high FSH levels, so this test will determine where your levels are.

- Karyotype. This test examines all forty-six chromosomes for abnormalities. Sometimes women with POF have only one X chromosome instead of two. There are other chromosomal disorders that are related to POF, which is why the karotype is useful.

- Luteinizing hormone (LH) test. In women with POF, LH levels are usually lower than FSH levels. This test will help determine where the levels are.

- Pregnancy test. This will rule out the possibility of an unexpected pregnancy.

- Serum estradiol (E2) test. Blood levels of E2 are usually lower in women who have POF.

- Thyroid studies. Optimal function of the thyroid is needed to make your sex hormones.

---

# Risk Factors for Both POD and POF

As mentioned, POD and POF are similar ailments. Consequently, they share a few common risk factors.

- Alcohol abuse
- Anorexia
- Bulimia
- Disruption of the hypothalamic-pituitary pathway
- Exposure to chemicals
- Exposure to radiation
- High altitudes
- Infections affecting the ovaries
- Malnutrition
- Medications, such as:
  Anticonvulsants
  Antidepressants
  Antipsychotics
- Mother smoked, consumed alcohol, or was around pesticides while pregnant
- Over-exercising
- Poor diet
- Recreational drug use
- Smoking
- Stress
- Thyroid disorders
- Weight issues (being over or underweight)

or she will likely also recommend you take progesterone in order to protect the lining of your uterus. Using these two hormones together can restart menstruation in women who may have stopped.

## DIAGNOSING POD AND POF

The gold standard to evaluate POD or POF, besides FSH and LH levels, is to have a twenty-eight-day salivary test done. This measures your levels of estrogen, progesterone, and testosterone throughout an entire month. Your DHEA, cortisol, and melatonin levels are also measured with this test, since they are also part of your hormonal symphony. This way, your healthcare practitioner will be able to develop a treatment program that is individualized to your own needs. No two women are alike, so the hormones you need at whichever stage in life you are at are unique to you.

# PREMATURE OVARIAN FAILURE (POF)

*See* Premature Ovarian Decline (POD).

# PREMENSTRUAL DYSPHORIC DISORDER (PMDD)

Premenstrual dysphoric disorder (PMDD) is a condition that is associated with severe emotional and physical symptoms that are linked to the menstrual cycle. PMDD is considered to be a severe form of PMS that affects about 5 to 10 percent of menstruating women.

PMDD is distinguished from PMS by the intensity and severity of its symptoms. The symptoms of PMDD are often so severe that they are considered disabling, meaning they get in the way of daily activities and relationships. By definition, the symptoms of PMDD start during the last week of your menstrual cycle and usually cease during the week following your cycle.

There are different types of PMDD. Some examples of PMDD are listed below.

- Symptoms start at mid-cycle (ovulation) and become worse as the cycle approaches and end shortly after the cycle begins.

- Symptoms start during the week before the menstrual cycle starts and end shortly after the cycle begins.

- Symptoms occur at ovulation and resolve after a few days but reoccur as the cycle approaches.

- Symptoms start at ovulation, become progressively worse, and continue until the menstrual cycle concludes.

Furthermore, these symptoms occur every month or almost every month.

## ▣ Symptoms of PMDD

The following are the symptoms that meet the criteria for the diagnosis of PMDD. The symptoms PMDD sufferers experience may change from month to month, but at least five of the following symptoms need to be present to make the diagnosis of PMDD.

☐ Difficulty concentrating and staying focused

☐ Fatigue, tiredness, or loss of energy

☐ Feeling out of control or overwhelmed

☐ Insomnia or sleeping too much

☐ Loss of interest in usual activities (work, school, or social activities)

☐ Marked anxiety, tension, or edginess

☐ Marked appetite change, overeating, or food cravings

☐ Persistent, marked irritability; anger; increased conflicts

☐ Physical symptoms such as weight gain, bloating, breast tenderness or swelling, headache, and muscle or joint pain

☐ Sudden mood swings (crying easily or extreme sensitivity)

☐ Very depressed mood, feeling hopeless

## Causes of PMDD

The cause of PMDD isn't clear. The current theories related to the cause of PMDD focus on the fact that it may not be due to a hormonal imbalance but rather to an imbalance of the neurotransmitters in your body. One neurotransmitter that is being looked at is serotonin, your "happy" neurotransmitter. Additionally, a number of women with severe PMS may have an underlying psychiatric disorder, and major depression is very common in women who have PMDD. However, PMDD can and does also occur in women who do not have depression.

## ■ Treating PMDD

PMDD treatment is designed to minimize or eliminate symptoms. Since symptoms vary, treatment will depend on the individual and the symptoms she is experiencing.

- Certain medications, such as:
  Anti-anxiety medications
  Diuretics (water pills)
  *Paxil CR* (parozetine controlled-release)
  YAZ (drospirenone ethinyl estradiol, an oral contraceptive)
  *Zoloft* (sertraline)
- Eating five to six small meals per day

- Exercise
- Increasing your complex carbohydrate and protein intake
- Limiting your intake of alcohol, caffeine, salt, and refined sugar
- Psychotherapy
- Hormonal therapy (usually progesterone, but testosterone and estrogen levels can be suboptimal)

## DIAGNOSING PMDD

In order to be diagnosed with PMDD, your symptoms must be severe enough to really disrupt your life. In other words, the symptoms interfere with work, school, relationships, and/or social activities.

### SUPPLEMENTATION TO TREAT PMDD

| Supplements | Dosage | Considerations |
|---|---|---|
| Calcium | 1,000 mg | |
| Chaste tree (vitex agnus castus) | Given as part of an herbal combination | |
| Vitamin $B_6$ | 100 mg | Take as part of a B complex vitamin with calcium and magnesium supplementation as well |

# PREMENSTRUAL SYNDROME (PMS)

Premenstrual syndrome (PMS) is a hormonal disorder that is characterized by the monthly recurrence of physical or psychological symptoms. It can be difficult to diagnose, because there are so many signs and symptoms associated with PMS. The only thing all the symptoms have in common is they all affect you only in the days before your monthly period. They usually subside when your menstrual cycle begins.

PMS affects between 60 and 75 percent of women in the United States, which means that as many as three of every four women who menstruate experience some form of PMS. The problems are more common in women who are between their late twenties and early forties. Generally, the problems and symptoms reoccur in predictable patterns, but some months may be more severe than others.

### ■ Symptoms of PMS

PMS has many symptoms associated with it. Some of these symptoms affect weight gain, such as abdominal bloating, appetite changes, and salt and sugar cravings. However, there are many other symptoms of PMS.

- ☐ Abdominal bloating
- ☐ Aches and pains
- ☐ Acne flare-ups
- ☐ Alcohol sensitivity
- ☐ Angry outbursts
- ☐ Anxiety
- ☐ Asthmatic attacks
- ☐ Avoidance of social activities
- ☐ Backache
- ☐ Bladder irritation
- ☐ Bleeding gums
- ☐ Breast tenderness
- ☐ Bruising
- ☐ Changes in appetite
- ☐ Clumsiness
- ☐ Confusion
- ☐ Conjunctivitis
- ☐ Constipation
- ☐ Cramps
- ☐ Craving salty foods or sweets
- ☐ Crying spells
- ☐ Decreased hearing
- ☐ Decreased productivity
- ☐ Decreased sex drive
- ☐ Depression
- ☐ Diarrhea or constipation
- ☐ Difficulty concentrating
- ☐ Dizziness
- ☐ Drowsiness
- ☐ Eye pain
- ☐ Facial swelling
- ☐ Fatigue
- ☐ Fear of going out alone
- ☐ Fear of losing control
- ☐ Food sensitivity
- ☐ Forgetfulness
- ☐ Headaches
- ☐ Herpes (cold sores)
- ☐ Hives or rashes
- ☐ Hot flashes
- ☐ Indecision
- ☐ Inefficiency
- ☐ Insomnia
- ☐ Irritability
- ☐ Joint pain
- ☐ Leg cramps
- ☐ Leg swelling
- ☐ Mood swings
- ☐ Muscle aches
- ☐ Nausea
- ☐ Palpitations
- ☐ Panic attacks
- ☐ Poor coordination
- ☐ Poor judgment
- ☐ Poor memory
- ☐ Poor vision
- ☐ Restlessness
- ☐ Ringing in ears
- ☐ Runny nose
- ☐ Seizures
- ☐ Sensitivity to light and noise
- ☐ Sinusitis
- ☐ Social withdrawal
- ☐ Sore throat
- ☐ Spots in front of eyes
- ☐ Suspiciousness
- ☐ Swollen fingers
- ☐ Tearfulness
- ☐ Tension
- ☐ Tingling in hands and feet
- ☐ Tremors
- ☐ Visual changes
- ☐ Vomiting
- ☐ Weight gain

Additionally, women with PMS tend to have low zinc levels. Zinc is involved in over 300 reactions in the body, including the production of the sex hormones. Thus, low zinc levels can lead to a host of problems including infertility, hypothyroidism, and elevated blood sugar levels.

The amount of symptoms may seem overwhelming, but in actuality, most women who have PMS experience only a few.

# Twenty-Eight-Day Menstrual Cycle

Every month, women who are of a reproductive age and who are not pregnant experience a menstrual cycle, which results in either pregnancy or menstruation. The average menstrual cycle is twenty-eight days long.

Days one to five of the cycle are considered the menstrual phase. The first day of a woman's period is considered the first day of the monthly menstrual cycle. If the egg has not been fertilized, it disintegrates. Low levels of estrogen and progesterone at this time cause the endometrium (the lining of the uterus) to break down and leave the body in the form of blood. This is known as a period, or a menstrual cycle. On average, the bleeding lasts about five days.

Expanding past the menstrual phase, days one to thirteen are considered the follicular phase. During this time, the brain releases follicle-stimulating hormone (FSH), which promotes the development of several follicles in the ovaries. Only one of these follicles, which each contain an egg, will reach maturity. As day thirteen approaches, the ovaries release more and more estrogen, thickening the uterine lining in case an egg gets fertilized.

Days ten to eighteen are the ovulatory phase. During this phase, the brain releases an abundance of luteinizing hormone (LH), which causes the mature follicle to bulge out from the surface of the ovary and burst, releasing the egg. This usually occurs around day fourteen. After this, the egg begins to travel down the fallopian tube and into the uterus. Fertilization, and therefore pregnancy, is most likely to occur during this phase.

Days fifteen to twenty-eight are the luteal phase. Having released the egg, the follicle develops into a corpus luteum, which secretes more and more progesterone, causing the endometrium to thicken further in case embryonic development takes place. If the egg is fertilized, the corpus luteum will begin to make human chorionic gonadotropin (HCG), which helps maintain the corpus luteum and its release of progesterone. Human chorionic gonadotropin is also the hormone that pregnancy tests detect.

The fertilized egg continues down the fallopian tube until it reaches the uterus, where it implants itself to the endometrium. This is where it develops into a fetus.

## ■ Causes of PMS

As of yet, the cause of PMS is not known. Changes in hormones during the menstrual cycle are definitely an important consideration. There are, however, several other theories and factors that contribute to PMS.

- Caffeine consumption.

- Low blood-sugar levels.

- Low estrogen levels. Estrogen levels change during your twenty-eight-day cycle, but not as dramatically as progesterone levels do. Your estrogen levels decrease at ovulation. They also decrease just before and during your cycle. When estrogen levels decline, your neurotransmitters change. Serotonin and dopamine levels decline, which can lead to depression. Also, when estrogen levels decrease, your norepinephrine levels may increase, which can make you feel more anxious and irritable.

- Low progesterone levels. Low progesterone levels on days twelve to fourteen of the menstrual cycle, which can be confirmed by saliva testing, are very commonly associated with PMS. There is no clear course of development when it comes to PMS. However, something in the person's life interferes with the pituitary-ovarian feedback loop, and it decreases the supply of progesterone.

- Oral contraceptives. Taking oral contraceptives may contribute to PMS, due to the progestin (synthetic progesterone) they contain.

- Partial hysterectomies. A partial hysterectomy may be a precipitating factor for PMS due to the decreased supply of blood to the ovaries post hysterectomy.

- Pregnancies, miscarriages, abortions, and tubal ligations (a procedure where the fallopian tubes are cut, burned, or blocked to prevent pregnancy) are also considered contributing factors to PMS. Studies have shown that after a tubal ligation, women have higher estrogen levels and lower progesterone levels in the second half of their cycle each month.

Additionally, some women who experience severe PMS symptoms have undiagnosed depression, but depression by itself does not cause all the PMS symptoms. Likewise, while stress can aggravate some symptoms, it does not cause them on its own.

Nutrition can also play a role. Deficiencies in certain vitamins and minerals, such as vitamin $B_6$, calcium, and magnesium, can make the symptoms of PMS worse. Eating a lot of salty foods can cause fluid retention, which can worsen symptoms. Drinking alcohol can cause mood and energy disturbances, which can also aggravate symptoms.

## ■ Treating PMS

There are many different ways to treat PMS, from medications and hormonal therapies, to nutrients and herbal modalities, to lifestyle changes. All have been shown to be effective. PMS can be treated with a success rate of more than 90 percent.

- Dietary adaptations. There are a few changes to your diet that can help decrease the PMS symptoms you are experiencing. Eating smaller meals more frequently can reduce bloating and fullness. Limiting your intake of salty foods can also reduce bloating. Avoiding caffeine and alcohol helps. Additionally, choosing fruits, vegetables, and whole grains (foods that are high in complex carbohydrates) and foods rich in calcium can help reduce PMS symptoms. Taking a multivitamin ensures you receive the nutrients you need, which can also help reduce PMS symptoms.

- Exercise. Exercising regularly can help reduce and manage PMS symptoms. Incorporating thirty minutes of exercise a day most days of the week can make a big difference. It can improve symptoms like fatigue and a depressed mood.

- Medications. There are a few medicines that doctors may prescribe for PMS symptoms. Medicines may work for some women and they may not help for others. The most commonly prescribed medications are

### DIAGNOSING PMS

There is no test to positively diagnose PMS. Doctors sometimes attribute symptoms to PMS based on your premenstrual pattern, which is established by keeping a record of your symptoms for at least two months (or however long your doctor requests). Show your record to your doctor, who will then determine the proper method of treatment.

# Menstrual Cramps

Menstrual cramps are dull or throbbing pains throughout the lower abdomen. They affect almost 50 percent of menstruating women just before and during their periods, making them one of the most common symptoms of PMS. The medical term for menstrual cramps is "dysmenorrhea." The pain tends to be intermittent; strongest in the lower part of the abdomen. But, it can also radiate to the back and inner thighs. Symptoms may go away after two or three hours, but they can last up to three days. The severity of symptoms also varies between women. For some, the pain is merely an annoyance and for others, it can get in the way of daily activities.

The cramps are classified into two categories: primary dysmenorrhea and secondary dysmenorrhea. Primary dysmenorrhea does not stem from a physical abnormality, but secondary dysmenorrhea is usually caused by endometriosis or uterine fibroids.

## Risk Factors for Menstrual Cramps

There are a few things that can contribute to menstrual cramps. Women who begin their cycles at younger ages (eleven or younger) and have longer menstrual periods tend to have more days of pain and increased severity. Additionally, all women under the age of twenty are at a higher risk for dysmenorrhea. Women who have never delivered a baby also have a greater chance of cramping. Heavy bleeding during periods can increase the risk of cramping. Being overweight doubles the risk of having long and painful cycles, but women between the ages of fourteen and twenty who try to lose weight may have a higher risk of menstrual cramps. Smoking, depression, and anxiety also increase the risk of cramping.

## Symptoms of Dysmenorrhea

The only symptom of dysmenorrhea is pain in the lower abdomen that sometimes radiates to the lower back and thighs. However, the cramping is sometimes accompanied by nausea, vomiting, loose stools, sweating, and dizziness.

## Causes of Dysmenorrhea

Elevated levels of prostaglandins (prostaglandin E2) may be one of the main causes of menstrual cramps. Studies have shown that women with dysmenorrhea produce eight to thirteen times more prostaglandin E2 than women who do not have painful cycles. High prostaglandin E2 levels may be associated with lower progesterone levels that occur in your body just before your cycle begins. Painful menstrual cycles occur only in cycles where you have ovulated because if you have not ovulated, no increase in progesterone occurs in the second part of the cycle.

## ■ Treating Dysmenorrhea

Treatment for dysmenorrhea can include any of the following methods:

- Acupuncture
- Biofeedback
- Homeopathy
- Prescription medications and/or nutritional therapies
- Therapeutic massage

There are some foods you should stay away from while you are cramping. Certain foods can aggravate your symptoms. Foods that are high in arachidonic acid will increase prostaglandin 2 and cause inflammation. Some of these foods are butter, corn and palm oils, coconut oil, soybean soils, and eggs. Any food that contains saturated fat such as beef, pork, and lamb should also be avoided. Turkey and chicken have less saturated fats than red meat, but contain more arachidonic acid. Eating any food that you are allergic to can also set up an inflammatory response and increase cramping. Wheat and dairy are very common allergens. For some women, salt may increase cramping.

The best foods to help alleviate cramping are those that increase prostaglandins 1 and 3. These prostaglandins are antispasmodic. Cold water fish such as salmon, tuna, halibut, and sardines, and flax and pumpkin seeds produce prostaglandins that relax muscle and decrease cramping. Sesame seeds and sunflower seeds also produce prostaglandins that decrease inflammation and cramping.

| SUPPLEMENTATION TO TREAT DYSMENORRHEA | | |
|---|---|---|
| **Supplements** | **Dosage** | **Considerations** |
| Calcium | 600 to 1000 mg | Helps decrease muscle tension. |
| EPA/DHA (fish oil) | 2,000 mg | Lowers prostaglandin 2 production and does not increase bleeding. |
| Magnesium | 300 to 500 mg | Helps decrease muscle tension. |
| Motherwort | Given as part of an herbal combination | Acts as an antispasmodic. |

| Niacin (vitamin B$_3$) | Use inside of B complex 100 mg | Taking vitamin C and rutin can help increase niacin's effectiveness. Take niacin seven to ten days before your cycle begins. |
| Progesterone | | Dosage depends on results of saliva or urine testing. |
| Pycnogenol | 30 mg, twice a day | Derived from the bark of a French maritime pine tree, and can also be found in grape seeds, chocolate, almonds, cranberries, and blueberries. |
| Vitamin E | 200 to 400 IU | Helps decrease cramping. |

Additionally, supplementation with valerian, crampbark, black haw, rose tea, and black cohosh can help ease the symptoms of cramps.

antidepressants, which help deal with fatigue and food cravings; non-steriodial anti-inflammatory drugs, which can ease cramping and breast discomfort; oral contraceptives, which help reduce physical and emotional side effects; diuretics, which can help you shed water weight; and Medroxyprogesterone acetate, an injection that can temporarily stop ovulation. However, in some cases it can also increase some PMS symptoms, so use with caution.

- Stress reduction. Making sure you get enough sleep is a good way to reduce stress, which can help alleviate PMS symptoms. Muscle relaxation exercises, deep breathing techniques, yoga, or massages are also good ways to reduce stress. (See section on cortisol and stress, page 35.)

## SUPPLEMENTATION TO TREAT PMS

| Supplements | Dosage | Considerations |
| --- | --- | --- |
| Angelica sinensis | Given as part of an herbal combination | Helps treat painful cycles (dysmenorrheal), absence of cycles (amenorrhea), and abnormal menstruation (metrorrhagia). Start supplementation on day fourteen of your cycle and continue until end of cycle. If you are taking it for abnormal cycles, stop before your cycle starts. |
| Borage oil | 500 to 1,000 mg | Can help reduce breast tenderness, fluid retention, cramps, and psychological PMS symptoms. |

| Calcium | 600 to 1,000 mg | Can help reduce breast tenderness, fluid retention, cramps, and psychological PMS symptoms. |
| --- | --- | --- |
| Evening primrose | 1,000 to 2,000 mg | Can help reduce breast tenderness, fluid retention, cramps, and psychological PMS symptoms. |
| Ginkgo biloba | 120 to 180 mg | Helps relieve breast pain and tenderness. |
| Licorice (glycyrrhiza glabra)* | Varies (see doctor for dosage) | Lowers estrogen levels and raises progesterone levels. Decreases water retention. Do not use if you have high blood pressure. |
| Magnesium | 300 to 600 mg | Can help reduce breast tenderness, fluid retention, cramps, and psychological PMS symptoms. |
| Omega-3 fatty acids | 1,000 to 2,000 mg | Can help reduce breast tenderness, fluid retention, cramps, and psychological PMS symptoms. |
| St. John's wort (Hypericum perforatum) | 500 mg twice a day | Do not take if you are on an antidepressant. |
| Taurine | 1,000 mg | Can help reduce breast tenderness, fluid retention, cramps, and psychological PMS symptoms. |
| Vitamin A | 5,000 to 8,000 IU (can use up to 25,000 IU under the direction of a physician) | Can help reduce breast tenderness, fluid retention, cramps, and psychological PMS symptoms. |
| Vitamin $B_6$ | 100 mg in a B complex | Can help reduce breast tenderness, fluid retention, cramps, and psychological PMS symptoms. |
| Vitamin $B_{12}$ | 1000 micrograms in a B complex | Can help reduce breast tenderness, fluid retention, cramps, and psychological PMS symptoms. |
| Vitamin E | 400 to 800 IU | Can help reduce breast tenderness, fluid retention, cramps, and psychological PMS symptoms. Do not use if you take Coumadin. |

* Licorice also blocks the hormone aldosterone, which decreases water retention. Many women who have bloating due to PMS have high aldosterone levels. Aldosterone helps regulate the sodium and potassium levels in the body. The main component of licorice is glycyrrhetinic acid, which binds to aldosterone receptors. Start licorice on day fourteen of your cycle and continue until your cycle commences. Do not use licorice if you have a history of hypertension (high blood pressure), since it may raise your pressure. Licorice is a pill and the amount that it can raise blood pressure is different in each person. Licorice should also not be used if you are taking the drug digitalis, a medication used to help the heart function more effectively.

Additionally, black cohosh and chasteberry have been proven useful for helping to ease PMS symptoms.

## Additional Treatments for PMS Symptoms

Since PMS is a state that is affected by low progesterone levels, progesterone supplementation has been found to be helpful. Supplementation should be with bio-identical progesterone, which is compounded to be the same chemical structure as the progesterone your body makes. This is also called natural progesterone. It is a prescription made by a compounding pharmacy to be used on days twelve to twenty-four (starting twelve days after your first day of bleeding) of the menstrual cycle. This progesterone is applied as a cream, which is derived from wild yams and soybeans. However, if you have insomnia, progesterone is best taken as a pill so that it affects the GABA receptors in the brain, which will produce a calming effect and allow you to sleep better. Otherwise, transdermally (on the skin) applied progesterone is usually used.

There is also a subset of women who have low estradiol (E2, a form of estrogen) levels and normal progesterone levels associated with PMS. For these women, progesterone supplementation will not work. Low levels of E2 are associated with neurotransmitter changes, including dopamine, norepinephrine, and epinephrine depletion. Furthermore, a rapid rise and fall in estrogen levels can affect serotonin production. This may trigger depression and changes in eating patterns. For this subset of women, the herbal therapies discussed previously may be more effective.

Phytoestrogens, also called dietary estrogens, have a very weak effect. They are only 2 percent as strong as estrogen so they do not replace estrogen. Phytoestrogens do, however, provide a balancing effect. If estrogen levels are high, they will decrease the effects of estrogen since they bind to estrogen receptor sites and compete with estrogen. If estrogen levels are low, phytoestrogens will increase the effects of estrogen.

Of course, you should always check with your healthcare professional before trying any of these remedies.

# ROSACEA

*See* Skin Problems.

# SKIN PROBLEMS

Your skin can be a good indicator of what is happening on the inside of your body. For example, it is hard for your skin to look smooth and soft if the remainder of your body has inflammation. Collagen, which helps keep your skin firm and strong, requires vitamin C to be made. Therefore, if your vitamin C levels are low, your skin may age. Additionally, imbalances of many hormones can be mirrored in your skin. You may have acne if your testosterone level is high. Conversely, if your testosterone levels are low you may have skin sagging. If your hormones are not balanced you may develop rosacea, an inflammatory skin condition.

## ▓ Some Causes of Skin Problems

- Depletion of essential fatty acids
- Emotional stress
- Excess of caffeine
- Food allergies
- Hormonal changes
- Inability of liver to detoxify
- Irritating cosmetics
- Leaky gut syndrome
- Low water consumption
- Refined foods and sugar
- Saturated fats

## ESTROGEN AND YOUR SKIN

Skin cells have estrogen receptors. As your estrogen levels start declining, there is a decrease in the elastin and collagen production in your connective tissue. Estrogens increase blood supply to your skin and improve the structure of elastic fibers. The amount of collagen in your skin is also maintained by estrogen and decreases after menopause. Collagen is very important to your skin. It serves as connective tissue between the cells and has many important functions in the body.

## ▓ Functions of Collagen in the Body

- Acts as a filler, making skin appear plumper and fuller
- Plays a role in tissue development
- Responsible for skin strength and elasticity
- Strengthens blood vessels
- Supports internal organs
- When hydrolyzed, can play a role in weight management

Furthermore, collagen is very susceptible to free radical damage, which can cause your skin to sag and to wrinkle by causing abnormal cross linking. This abnormal cross linking causes your skin to be stiff and unable to retain water and remain plump.

In addition to maintaining collagen, estrogen increases the water content of your skin by increasing the production of hyaluronic acid. Hyaluronic acid is a large sugar molecule that is rich in collagen. It attracts and binds water. Your body's hyaluronic acid content declines with age due to free radical damage and estrogen loss. Hyaluronic acid also makes your skin look soft and contributes to your skin's thickness. So, if you are sixty years old and you are not taking estrogen, your skin will be only about half as thick as women the same age who do take estrogen.

Estrogen also helps your skin look younger by maintaining its firmness. Recent studies have shown that topical estrogens, such as estriol (E3), have improved elasticity and firmness of the skin and decreased wrinkle depth and pore size by 61 to 100 percent. In my office, we use E3 topically compounded with antioxidants. You will need a prescription for this.

Declining levels of testosterone, progesterone, and growth hormone also contribute to the wrinkling of your skin.

Likewise, if you want your skin to look younger, do not use petroleum-based products. Look out also for products containing mineral oil. Mineral oil is a mixture of refined liquid carbohydrates derived from petroleum, and it is used as a stabilizing ingredient in many skin formulas.

### ■ Problems With Petroleum-Based Products

• Block water and nutrients so they cannot be absorbed.

• Cannot be absorbed by the skin and are foreign to its cellular structure.

• Decrease perspiration, which is needed to allow your body to detoxify, by 40 to 60 percent.

• Dry out your skin by removing the fine coating of sebum normally found on the surface of your skin.

## AGING AND YOUR SKIN

As your body ages it produces less energy needed for cell regeneration and the repair of DNA. Your supply of antioxidants also declines. Oxidation causes the fatty membranes of your cells to become more permeable, which causes you to lose moisture. Your skin will become dehydrated, and this causes your skin to age. The aging process also causes a decrease in your body's ability to stay moisturized due to a decline in the making of essential fatty acids. Therefore, it is important to take omega-3-fatty acids like fish oil on a daily basis to keep your skin hydrated. Your skin also loses moisture with age due to a decline in sodium pyrrolidone carboxylic acid which helps your skin stay hydrated by absorbing water from the air. After the age of fifty, the level of sodium pyrrolidone carboxylic acid decreases by one-half.

Age spots are due to melanocytes clumping together, which makes the skin appear to have brown spots. Skin-lightening agents such as n-acetyl glucosamine and niacinamide have been shown to be very effective in the treatment of age spots. When they are used together they stimulate the production of hyaluronic acid. Both of these agents can be added to your customized skin care creams.

## ■ Other Nutrients That Are Important for Youthful Skin

- Alpha lipoic acid decreases glycation so that your skin is smoother and firmer. It also stimulates activating protein-1, which, if activated by alpha lipoic acid, turns on enzymes that digest your damaged collagen.

- Coenzyme Q-10 is needed by your body to help the fibroblasts produce collagen and elastin. As you age, the mitochondria (engines of the cells) begin to dysfunction in the fibroblasts. This makes the fibroblasts less able to produce energy needed to support the skin. This decrease in energy contributes to the visible signs of skin aging. Applying coenzyme Q-10 to your skin helps to replenish levels in the skin cells, which decreases some of the causes of skin wrinkling and sagging.

- DMAE (dimethylaminoethanol) helps to keep your skin from sagging by stabilizing your cell membranes. It also helps increase the radiance, tone, and firmness of your skin along with decreasing inflammation. DMAE has an odor that needs to be masked if it is applied to the skin.

- Pomegranate seed oil extract helps to promote the regeneration and thickening of your skin.

- Red tea extract is a strong antioxidant, which decreases inflammation.

- Vitamin E. The alpha-tocopherol form decreases skin roughness and the depth of wrinkles when applied to your skin.

Your Metabolic/Anti-Aging specialist can write a prescription to compound nutrients and, if needed, estriol to make your own personalized skin care program that is applied transdermally. When it comes to skin care, one size does not fit all. You deserve a personalized approach to your anti-aging skin care program.

## STRESS

*See* Heart Disease; Osteoporosis; Polycystic Ovarian Syndrome (PCOS); Postpartum Depression; Skin Problems.

## STROKE

*See* Heart Disease.

## STRONTIUM DEFICIENCY

*See* Osteoporosis.

## SURGICAL MENOPAUSE

*See* Menopause.

## URINARY LEAKAGE

*See* Bladder Problems.

## UTERINE CANCER

*See* Cancer.

## VAGINAL ISSUES

*See* Menopause; Premature Ovarian Decline (POD); Vulvodynia.

## VAGINITIS

*See* Diethylstilbestrol (DES) Babies.

## VITAMIN C DEFICIENCY

*See* Skin Problems.

## VITAMIN D DEFICIENCY

*See* Osteoporosis.

## VOMITING

*See* Premenstrual Syndrome (PMS).

## VULVODYNIA

Vulvodynia is the medical term for vaginal pain. Low estrogen levels can result in vaginal burning that can become so painful that intercourse may become impossible. Estrogen cream or suppositories used vaginally have been shown to be helpful for many people. The vaginal cream may have to be made by a compounding pharmacist in the same manner natural hormone replacement is made, because you may have burning and increased pain due to the preservative in commercially-available prescription vaginal creams. For some women, low testosterone levels may also be a contributing factor to vulvodynia. Testosterone cream can be mixed with estrogen made by the compounding pharmacy.

For some women, food triggers an attack of vulvodynia. Foods that contain chemicals such as citric acid, salicylic acid, and oxalates may increase pain related to vulvodynia. The following is a list of foods that have been implicated as triggers for vulvodynia.

- Alcohol
- Apples
- Bananas
- Caffeine (coffee, tea, carbonated beverages with caffeine)

- Chemical preservatives
- Chocolate
- Citrus foods
- Dyes that contain tartrazine
- Lentils
- Lima beans
- Sharp cheeses
- Spicy food
- Sweeteners (aspartame, saccharin)
- Tobacco
- Tomatoes
- Yogurt

Preservatives in foods and even medications may present a problem if you have vulvodynia. PEG is a preservative that is put in the cream to keep it sterile. This can be used in non-compounding or even compounding pharmacies, so the physician needs to specify whether or not PEG is being used when the vaginal cream is being made by the compounding pharmacy.

## WEIGHT GAIN

*See* Menopause; Polycystic Ovarian Syndrome (PCOS); Premenstrual Dysphoric Disorder (PMDD); Premenstrual Syndrome (PMS).

## ZINC DEFICIENCY

*See* Osteoporosis; Premenstrual Syndrome (PMS).

# PART III

# Hormone Replacement Therapy

# Introduction to Part III

**A** woman's body is designed to not need hormonal therapy. If you are nutritionally sound, not stressed, you exercise, you are not overweight, and you are not toxic, your body will usually make the right amount of hormones before and after menopause. However, in today's world there are very few women who fall into this category.

The good news is we now have the science to balance the hormones in your body—no matter what age you are. Whether you are suffering from PMS, PCOS, or postpartum depression (which are all caused by hormonal imbalances), balancing your hormones is a key component to help you feel great. If you are infertile, optimizing and balancing your hormonal levels may help you conceive. Additionally, if you are perimenopausal or menopausal, balancing your hormones will not only help you relieve symptoms—it will also decrease your risk of developing other diseases.

The great news is that you can now have your hormone replacement therapy individualized and customized to meet your own personal needs. In the past, the only type of hormonal therapy available was a "one-size-fits-all" type, which meant that every woman, regardless of symptoms and severity of symptoms, received the same dosage of hormonal treatment. This is a problem, as you may know, since two women with similar symptoms may have two entirely different ailments. Now, with customizable hormonal therapy, this is no longer the case. Women can receive treatment specifically designed for their body and symptoms.

In this part of the book, you will learn what HRT is. The difference between synthetic and natural hormonal replacement therapy will be explained, along with studies that show why natural HRT may be the better option. Reasons you should consider HRT and information on how to get started once you have decided to do so are also provided. Different types of tests that measure hormonal levels are detailed in this part of the book as well.

Additionally, Part III will discuss a few examples of HRT and how proper nutrition and herbal remedies can alleviate symptoms and maximize your treatment.

Welcome to the new era of medicine.

# WHAT IS HRT?

Up until a few decades ago, the only hormonal therapy available in this country was synthetic hormone replacement.

## SYNTHETIC HRT

Some people may hear the word "synthetic" and think "fake," but this is not always the case. When it comes to hormone replacement, the word synthetic means "not the same chemical structure that your own body makes." On the contrary, "natural," when referring to hormones, means "the exact same chemical structure as what your body makes." It does not necessarily mean that the item has a plant origin, even though hormones are made from soy or yams.

If the chemical structure of the hormone matches the chemical structure of the hormone in your body, it is called "bio-identical." Therefore, even though some hormones are produced in a laboratory, they are still called natural and bio-identical if they match the chemical structure in your body. Anything else is called synthetic.

The government-sponsored Women's Health Initiative Program halted its study on estrogen plus progestin (synthetic progesterone, or Prempro) on July 9, 2002. The study was conducted on 16,000 women who had not had a hysterectomy. Participants were either given Prempro or a placebo. The study was ended three years earlier than initially planned because researchers found that there was an increased risk of breast cancer in some of the women who were participating in the study and taking the hormones. Analysis of the study also revealed that heart attack risk began increasing in the progestin group early in the study.

The study revealed that the women taking Prempro, when compared to the women taking the placebo, had:

• A 22 percent increase in heart disease.

• A 24 percent decrease in total fracture rate.

• A 26 percent increase in breast cancer development.

• A 33 percent decrease in fracture rate of the hip.

• A 37 percent decrease in colorectal cancer.

- A 41 percent higher risk of stroke.

- Double the rate of blood clots.

Additional studies, such as the Heart and Estrogen/Progestin Replacement Study Follow-Up (HERS II), agree with the findings of the Women's Health Initiative Program. HERS II results also showed an increase in cardiovascular risk for the women taking synthetic progesterone. Likewise, several other studies have shown recently that progestins (synthetic progesterone) have an unfavorable effect on cholesterol levels and may promote cardiovascular disease.

Furthermore, a recent Danish medical trial has shown a link between synthetic hormone replacement and an increased risk of developing ovarian cancer. The elevated risk depends on which hormones are used, how long the person takes them, and the route of administration.

## Other Problems With Synthetic HRT

Synthetic HRT has also been shown to have other problems:

- It is estimated that one-half of women quit taking their synthetic hormone replacement therapy after one year because they are unable to tolerate the side effects.

- Synthetic hormones waste energy by giving incomplete messages to cells, which then fail to produce a balanced hormonal response.

The results of the Women's Health Initiative Study brought to the forefront why synthetic hormonal therapy will quickly become a treatment of the past. A groundbreaking article by Dr. Kent Holtorf was published in the medical journal *Postgraduate Medicine* in January 2009. Dr. Holtorf's article answered the question of whether natural hormones are safer or more efficacious than synthetic hormones. After an extensive review of medical literature, the article concluded that the "physiological data and clinical outcomes demonstrate that bioidentical hormones are associated with lower risks, including the risk of breast cancer and cardiovascular disease, and are more efficacious than their synthetic and animal-derived counterparts. Until evidence is found to the contrary, bioidentical hormones remain the preferred method of HRT."

In the following pages you will discover the answer to HRT: customized natural (bio-identical) hormone replacement that is available as a prescription (not over-the-counter). As Joseph Collins, ND, author of *What's Your Menopause Type?* puts it: "Today's truth is this: There is no magic hormone or combination of hormones that can be indiscriminately used by all women. Each woman is an individual and hormonal balance must be the ultimate goal for all women."

## NATURAL HRT

The results of the Women's Health Initiative Study (see page 157 for more information) highlight the problems associated with "one size fits all" hormone replacement, which is when all women suffering hormonal problems—regardless of their symptoms—are instructed to take the same type and dosage of hormones. What is needed is for doctors to more carefully evaluate each woman's own unique set of environmental, genetic, and physiological risk factors to determine a HRT plan that is designed to fit her individual needs. For this, there is natural hormone replacement.

If you are taking natural hormone replacement, it means you are using hormones that are biologically identical to, or the same chemical structure as, the ones your body makes.

One size does *not* fit all. Customized natural hormonal therapy is the best way to replace hormones safely. The reason for this is because your hormone response is as unique to you as your fingerprints are. How a woman responds to HRT is related to her genetic profile, stress level, health condition, environment, nutritional supplementation, and diet. Since no two women share the same lifestyle, it goes without saying that no two women will share the same HRT therapy.

### ■ Six Reasons You Should Consider HRT

1. Bone production (prevention of osteoporosis).

2. Growth and repair.

3. Heart health.

4. Prevention of memory loss.

5. Relief of symptoms related to any/all of the issues discussed in Part II.

6. Studies have shown that women who use hormone replacement live longer than those who do not.

## Compounded Hormones

The way to ensure you get the HRT you need is to use compounded hormones. With compounded hormones, your HRT therapy will be made for your own individual needs. Your doctor can have a compounding pharmacist make your prescription for you and you only. Your HRT will be made from plant extractions that are an exact replica of your own hormones.

The key to effective hormone replacement therapy, in summary, is individuality. Fixed doses do not allow for customized, tailor-made treatment. Having your hormonal therapy customized at any age helps maintain the optimal hormonal symphony for your body.

## CONSIDERATIONS

If you are considering HRT, you should make sure you thoroughly understand how all of your body's hormones work and interact with each other. For example, insulin resistance and hyperinsulinemia (elevated insulin levels) influence the synthesis of testosterone and the metabolism of DHEA in women. Therefore, insulin resistance is involved with increased testosterone levels and depletion of DHEA. This occurs because the increase in insulin elevates the activity of an enzyme, 17, 20-lyase, which converts DHEA to cortisol and testosterone. This encourages obesity.

To take this concept one step further, a study done at the University of Toronto revealed a 283 percent increase in the risk of breast cancer in women with elevated insulin levels. This is because there are insulin receptors on breast cells. Cancer cells also have insulin receptors. Insulin attaches to the receptor and turns it on, which increases the growth of cancer cells. Therefore, if your blood sugar is high you may be increasing your risk of breast and other kinds of cancer.

## GETTING STARTED ON HRT

The good news is that the science is here to help. You can have this individualized kind of medical care. Make sure that you see a fellowship trained, master's degree specialist in Metabolic/Anti-Aging Medicine. These specifications guarantee your healthcare practitioner has completed an extra two to three years of training in natural hormonal therapies.

For information on how to find this type of specialist, see the Resources section (page 183).

# HORMONAL TESTING METHODS

You should have your hormone levels measured before you begin hormone replacement therapy, no matter what age you are. There are a few different methods you can use to get your hormonal levels measured.

## SALIVARY TESTING

Salivary, or saliva, testing is the preferred method of hormone testing for perimenopausal women, menopausal women, and women with PMS symptoms or other hormonal imbalances.

Salivary testing is also an excellent way to evaluate infertility, since a twenty-eight-day test can be done. This test gives your doctor the ability to look at your estrogen, progesterone, and testosterone levels throughout your entire monthly cycle. Many times stress plays a role in infertility and the twenty-eight-day saliva test also measures your cortisol and DHEA levels.

Saliva testing measures only the "free" form of the hormones. (On the contrary, having your blood levels measured will tell you the amount of free and bound hormones in your body.) This is important because the free hormone molecules are the only ones available for your body to use. (Bound hormones are stored, and not available for immediate use.) Saliva testing measures levels throughout your entire body. Measuring the hormone levels throughout your body is crucial. Not doing so can result in an incorrect prescription.

There are hormone receptors all over the body. For example, there are not only estrogen receptors in the breast and gonadal tissues, but also in the eyes. Saliva testing is also the optimal way to measure hormone levels because it allows for changes over a number of days, as opposed to a one-time blood draw that shows levels only at the time of the test.

Hormone level measurement should be repeated about three months after you begin hormone replacement therapy. Subsequently, tests should then be done on a routine basis depending on your own personal needs (your healthcare practitioner should advise you as to what these are). Salivary testing will help your healthcare practitioner better maintain the level of hormone replacement that is right for you.

## TWENTY-FOUR-HOUR URINE TESTS

Twenty-four-hour urinary testing of hormonal function is also an accurate method of measuring hormone levels and hormonal function. Urine testing is able to measure the hormone level over time and, like saliva testing, evaluates the amount of free hormones. Urine testing also measures hormone levels throughout the whole body. It is also able to measure the downstream metabolites, or breakdown products, of the sex hormones, which include many circulating estrogens in the body as well as other breakdown products. This is advantageous because it helps to make sure the hormones are broken down into metabolites that decrease the risk of disease and not increase the risk of other pathological processes. Hormones in the urine are reflective of the combination of both endocrine production and peripheral production of the hormones and their metabolites. In other words, urinary hormones tell your doctor the hormone levels produced by your hormonal system and also your hormone production and conversion that occurs throughout your entire body. Urinary hormones are also a good method to look at the wear and tear (catabolic) versus the rest and recovery (anabolic) balance in the body. If you are in optimal health, your anabolic state is higher than your catabolic state. A high catabolic state ages you because your body is spending more time breaking down than building up your metabolism. Do not overhydrate if you are taking a urine hormone test because it can affect the accuracy of the testing.

## BLOOD TESTS

One kind of blood test is the SHBG test. This test measures your levels of sex hormone binding globulin (SHBG).

SHBG is a glycoprotein that binds to testosterone and estradiol. (Progesterone and cortisol bind to transcortin.) Once bound to SHBG, testosterone and estradiol circulate in the bloodstream. Only a small amount of testosterone and estradiol is left unbound or free. This unbound part is biologically active and able to enter a cell and activate its receptor. SHBG decreases testosterone and estrogen's ability to do this. Therefore, the availability of your sex hormones is related to SHBG.

SHBG is produced by your liver and then released into your bloodstream. The brain, uterus, vagina, and placenta also produce SHBG. The amount of SHBG that is produced is regulated by other hormones in your body. For example, if your insulin level is too high the amount of SHBG produced is lower. In other words, if your body is producing too much insulin (as is the case with insulin resistance and type-2 diabetes) then you have more estrogen and testosterone available as free hormones for the body to use because there is less SHBG available for these hormones to bind to. Another example of the hormonal interplay that occurs with SHBG is that elevated testosterone levels decrease SHBG and high estrogen and thyroxine (one of the thyroid hormones) levels increase SHBG levels. Recent studies have shown that an elevated level of SHBG may be associated with an increase in breast cancer risk.

## ■ Medical Conditions Associated With SHBG Deficiency

- Diabetes
- Hypothyroidism
- PCOS

## ■ Medical Conditions Associated With SHBG Excess

- Anorexia nervosa
- Hyperthyroidism
- Pregnancy

Blood testing is also used to measure thyroid hormones and insulin.

A study showed that 45 percent of women on estrogen had suboptimal levels to maintain their memory and bone structure when their doctor went by symptoms only and did not measure hormone levels. This led researchers to conclude that monitoring symptoms alone was not enough. Therefore, repeated measurement of your hormone levels is needed in order for your doctor to optimize your hormone replacement therapy. Estrogen, progesterone, testosterone, cortisol, and DHEA are all hormones and should not be prescribed without measuring levels first and then on a regular basis. (See the Resources section on page 183 for availability of testing.)

Hormones do not function by themselves. As you have been learning, they are a symphony, a web that is inter-related. Measuring the metabolites of your sex hormones reveals enzyme activity and facilitates a deeper level of intervention to individualize and customize your care.

# Herbal Therapies for Hormonally-Related Symptoms

Herbal supplements are wonderful to help resolve symptoms like hot flashes and night sweats. However, they may not be enough to maintain your bone structure, prevent heart disease, or help you maintain your memory. *Do not use any of the herbs in this section if you are pregnant, nursing, or if you have been diagnosed with breast cancer. All of these herbs can interfere with the efficacy of birth control pills and HRT.*

## BLACK COHOSH (CIMICIFUGA RACEMOSA)

### ■ Functions of Black Cohosh

- Acts as a sedative
- Acts as an anti-inflammatory
- Acts as an anti-spasmotic
- Has a balancing effect on estrogen (if you have too much estrogen, black cohosh lowers it and if estrogen is too low, it enhances estrogen's effects)
- Has a direct effect on the hypothalamus (brain) to decrease hot flashes
- Is a relaxant
- Lowers blood pressure
- Lowers LDL (bad) cholesterol
- May relieve mild depression
- Relieves muscle soreness

### ■ Contraindications

- Do not take black cohosh if you are taking an antidepressant or have breast cancer

### ■ Side Effects of Black Cohosh

- Diarrhea
- Dizziness
- Headaches
- Impaired circulation
- Nausea
- Vertigo
- Vomiting

## CHASTEBERRY (VITEX AGNUS CASTUS)

### ■ Functions of Chasteberry

- Acts as a diuretic (water pill)
- Decreases LH and prolactin
- Raises progesterone and facilitates progesterone function

### ■ Contraindications

- Do not take if you have breast cancer
- May interfere with dopamine antagonist medications

## DONG QUAI (ANGELICA ARCHANGELICA)
### ■ Functions of Dong Quai

- Contains phytoestrogens

### ■ Contraindications

- Do not take if you have breast cancer
- Do not use if you have the cold or flu
- Do not use if you have diarrhea
- Interacts with anti-coagulants (blood thinners)
- May make menstrual blood flow heavier so do not use if your cycles are already heavy

# SELECTIVE ESTROGEN RECEPTOR MODULATORS (SERMS)

Selective estrogen receptor modulators (SERMS) are a type of hormone replacement therapy (HRT). An estrogen receptor is a group of receptors in your body that is activated by the hormone estrogen. Estrogen effects are mediated through two different estrogen receptors called estrogen receptor-alpha and estrogen receptor-beta. Estrogen receptor-alpha increases breast cell proliferation (growth). Estrogen receptor-beta inhibits (decreases) cell growth and prevents breast cancer development.

Some estrogen receptor modulators, such as estriol (E3), are made inside your body. These are called endogenous estrogen receptor modulators. There are also exogenous estrogen receptor modulators which are made from external sources like plants (phytoestrogens) and pharmaceutical medications like tamoxifen.

SERMs work by blocking the effects of estrogen in your breast tissue. They remain inside your estrogen receptors in your breast cells, preventing estrogen from entering and attaching to the cell. This stops the cell from receiving estrogen's signal to grow and multiply.

Of course, the cells in your body's other tissues also have estrogen receptors, which are all structured slightly differently depending on what cell they are in. Since SERMs are selective, as their name informs, they only block estrogen from one type of cell—the breast tissue cell. However, SERMs can activate estrogen's action in other cells.

## TYPES OF SERMS

There are three types of SERMs: tamoxifen, raloxifene, and toremifene. They are all taken in pill form.

### Tamoxifen

Tamoxifen (brand name *Nolvadex*) is given to women who have had cancer to help prevent a recurrence. It works by blocking estrogen's effects on your breast tissue since it occupies the cellular receptor sites for estrogen. However, tamoxifen does not block estrogen's affects elsewhere in your body—only on your breast tissues. Consequently, it can double or triple your risk of cancer of the uterus. It also increases your risk of blood clots.

### Raloxifene

Raloxifene (brand name *Evista*) is also a SERM. It has selective estrogen activity for bones, which means it helps maintain bone structure and therefore decreases the risk of osteoporosis. It has been shown to decrease your risk for breast cancer. Raloxifene can increase bone density up to 20 percent. A side effect of raloxifene is hot flashes.

### Toremifene

Toremifene (brand name *Fareston*) is used to treat post-menopausal women who have been disgnosed with advanced hormone-receptor-positive breast cancer.

SERMs decrease total cholesterol by 5 percent and LDL (bad cholesterol) by 10 percent. However, they are not very effective in lowering triglycerides and they do not increase HDL (good cholesterol) as well as synthetic or natural hormone replacement therapy do. Furthermore, the designer estrogens, raloxifene (*Evista*) and tamoxifen (*Nolvadex*), are not neuroprotective for the brain. Consequently, they will not have the same positive effect on your memory and mood as natural estrogen does. (For more on natural estrogens, see page 8.)

# BIRTH CONTROL PILLS

What a woman should choose as a birth control method is always an interesting discussion. Nutritional depletions, like the ones discussed in this section, are one of the key issues. If you are going to take birth control pills, it is important that you supplement with a pharmaceutical-grade multivitamin to replace the nutrients that are depleted with this kind of medication.

Birth control pills can have the following effects on your body:

- Birth control pills can deplete your body of zinc and can elevate copper levels in your system. This can have many side effects, including abdominal pain, anemia, diarrhea, fatigue, headaches, memory impairment, and sleep disturbances.

- Birth control pills contain progestin (synthetic progesterone). As you have seen in the section on progesterone (page 19), progestin use can make the symptoms of a progesterone deficiency worse. Likewise, progestins decrease the protective effects of estrogen on your heart.

- Estrogen-containing birth control pills decrease vitamins $B_6$, $B_{12}$, and folate in your body. These vitamins are needed to metabolize homocysteine, an amino acid. A buildup of homocysteine in your body can predispose you to heart disease, Alzheimer's disease, or depression.

- Even low-dose birth control pills contain more estrogens and progestin than the amount that is usually needed for treatment of perimenopause or menopause.

- Women taking birth control pills have been shown to have decreased serum testosterone and DHEA levels.

For all of the above reasons, birth control pills may not be the optimal HRT for perimenopausal and menopausal women.

# NUTRITION AND HRT

Proper nutrition plays an important part in maximizing your HRT, preventing disease, and general treatment of menopause.

The following nutrients and supplements can help you deal with hormonally-related symptoms.

| SUPPLEMENTATION TO HELP MAXIMIZE HRT | | |
|---|---|---|
| Supplements | Dosage | Considerations |
| Boron | 1 mg | Increases testosterone and decreases calcium loss in bones. |
| Fiber | 30 to 50 g | Decreases your cancer risk by decreasing estrogen levels in the blood. If you are estrogen dominant this is a good thing. |
| Folate | 800 micrograms | Repairs DNA and lowers breast cancer risk. |
| Vanadium | 10 to 50 mg | A deficiency can increase progesterone, but too much can decrease progesterone, so levels should always be at a healthy balance. |
| Vitamin A | 5,000 to 8,000 IU | Helps make hormones. |
| Vitamin C | 1,000 to 2,000 mg | Helps make hormones. |
| Vitamin E | 400 IU, twice a day | Helps relieve hot flashes. Also protects adrenals and ovaries from free radical damage. |
| Zinc | 25 to 50 mg | Makes your sex hormones, helps make healthy breast tissue, promotes ovarian and adrenal gland function, and maximizes estrogen receptor function. |

# Conclusion

The science of medicine in today's world is maturing. The previous concept that one agent causes a single disease and is treated with one medication is no more. Now, medicine has progressed into a deeper understanding of the complexities of human beings—women specifically, for the purpose of this text.

I hope that this book has shown you that medicine today looks at each individual molecule. It looks at cellular messengers and intercellular communication, which work to coordinate function between different organ systems. This paradigm shift in medicine is exemplified in the hormonal symphony in the body. Your hormonal needs are not stagnant; they change throughout your lifetime. They are affected by age, pregnancies, medications, exercise, toxins, and even your spiritual belief system. Hormonal needs also vary on a person-to-person basis. Consequently, you will need different hormones in different amounts throughout your life—even if you are experiencing similar symptoms as another woman, your hormonal needs may differ.

The Human Genome Project has helped us understand the biochemical individuality of medicine. One size does not fit all. This personalization of care is achievable through a functional approach to healthcare connected to the newest and fastest growing medical subspecialty: Metabolic/Anti-Aging medicine. This specialty looks at the cause of the problem instead of treating only the symptoms. With the realization in medicine that approximately 20 percent of disease is inherited and 80 percent is the environment that you put your body in, Metabolic/Anti-Aging medicine illustrates the importance of helping you, the patient, maintain a healthy terrain in your body. The goal is abatement of your symptoms that you thought were part of your normal physiologic landscape.

Your hormones function as a web. The right levels of all of your hormones are needed for you to be healthy. Hormone restoration and balance can play an integral role in helping you achieve optimal health.

To get in touch with Dr. Smith, please contact the Center for Healthy Living at 1-866-960-0178 or go to www.cfhll.com.

# Summaries

This section was designed to be a quick reference guide for the material included in this book. Important points have been pulled out and organized into a bulleted list.

## PART I: HORMONES

### Estrogen

- Your body has receptor sites for estrogen everywhere: in your brain, muscles, bone, bladder, gut, uterus, ovaries, vagina, breasts, eyes, heart, lungs, and blood vessels, to name a few.

- Estrogen has over 400 crucial functions in your body. You need optimal estrogen levels to be healthy.

- The amount of estrogen you have is important. Levels that are too low or too high can lead to symptoms or disease.

- Your body makes three main estrogens:

  Estrone (E1). Many researchers believe E1 may be related to an increase in breast cancer.

  Esradiol (E2). E2 helps maintain your memory, bone health, and aids in protecting you from heart disease.

  Estriol (E3). Considerable evidence exists to show that E3 may protect against breast cancer.

- Synthetic estrogen is not the same chemical structure of the estrogen that your body makes. Therefore, synthetic estrogen does not fit into the estrogen receptors in your body.

- Synthetic estrogens take a long time to be eliminated from your system.

- The preferred method for the administration of estrogen is transdermally (applied to the skin). Be sure to rub it in for two minutes.

- Estrogen synthesis, estrogen metabolism, and estrogen detoxification are of paramount importance in order to maintain optimal health.

- Diet affects estrogen production and use of estrogen.

- Have your Metabolic/Anti-Aging specialist measure all three types of estrogens before you start HRT.

- It is important for optimal health that your HRT be comprised of E2 and E3 (bi-est) and that it does *not* contain E1. E2 alone may be too strong an estrogen to use as hormone replacement. Plus, when you use E2 only, the protective affects of E3 are not present.

- How you metabolize estrogen is important.

- The 2-hydroxy estrogens are believed to be the "good estrogens" and are suggested to be anti-cancerous.

- The 16- and 4-hydroxy estrogens are believed to be associated with an increased risk of breast cancer.

- Equine estrogens, such as Premarin, increase 4-hydroxy estrogens.

- Diet, nutrients, and moderate exercise can increase your good estrogens. If you are undernourished and lacking key vitamins or nutrients, you may not be able to break down estrogen properly.

- The effect of estrogen on your body is not related solely to its synthesis and metabolism, but also to how it is detoxified. It is very important for you to detoxify estrogen completely in your body.

- Consuming foods high in indole-3-carbinol (or taking supplementation of this nutrient) is one of the best ways to increase good estrogen production.

- See a Metabolic/Anti-Aging specialist to have your estrogen metabolism test done.

- Estrogen has many protective effects on your brain.

- Estrogen helps maintain your memory and cognitive function. It also increases your ability to learn new things.

- Women on estrogen are less then half as likely to get Alzheimer's disease then women who are not on estrogen. Furthermore, estrogen use in post-menopausal women may delay the start of Alzheimer's disease.

- Salivary testing or a twenty-four hour urine test are the preferred methods of measuring your levels of estrogen.

## Progesterone

- Progesterone plays a role in ovulation, menstruation, and pregnancy.

- Unlike excess estrogen, which can be caused by a variety of factors, high progesterone levels can only result if a woman is taking too much progesterone or too much pregnenolone.

- Natural progesterone is a hormone that helps with your mood. Anxiety, irritability, insomnia, mood swings, and depression, as well as many other symptoms, are helped by natural progesterone.

- Synthetic progesterone, called progestin, has many side effects and does not function the same way in your body as natural progesterone. Progestins do not reproduce the actions of natural progesterone.

- Progestins stop the protective effects of estrogen on your heart. Natural progesterone is synergistic and increases the protective affects of estrogen on your heart.

- The use of synthetic progesterone increases the risk of breast cancer by 800 percent when compared to the use of estrogen alone.

- If you have had a hysterectomy, you may still need progesterone.

- It is important that you have your levels of progesterone measured before you begin HRT and then on a regular basis to confirm that you remain on an optimal dose afterwards.

- Stress increases adrenaline, which can block progesterone receptors and prevent progesterone from being used effectively in your body.

- If you take only progesterone and not estrogen (and your body is deficient in estrogen) this may predispose you to diabetes.

- If you have insomnia, choose the pill form of progesterone, which will help you sleep better than progesterone applied to your skin.

- Natural progesterone offers a safer approach to HRT than synthetic progesterone does.

- Salivary testing or a twenty-four hour urine test are the preferred methods of measuring your levels of progesterone.

## Estrogen/Progesterone Ratio

- Estrogen and progesterone work together in your body. It is important that estrogen and progesterone remain in a specific ratio within your body.

- There is a higher risk for breast cancer if you have a low progesterone-to-estrogen ratio, which means that the estrogen and progesterone ratio in your body is out of balance.

## Testosterone

- Testosterone falls into a class of hormones called "androgens." Androgens are commonly referred to as "male" hormones, but they are present in women.

- Testosterone should be given *with* estrogen. If given alone, testosterone can increase your risk of heart disease if your body no longer has enough estrogen. Estrogen is needed to help testosterone work.

- As women go through menopause, about 20 percent of them will experience high testosterone levels that will not decline with age.

- Synthetic testosterone has been linked to cancer of the liver.

- Excessive testosterone can cause symptoms and increase your risk of obesity, diabetes, and heart disease.

- Dihydrotestosterone (DHT) is a byproduct of testosterone. High DHT levels can cause hair loss in women.

- Salivary testing or a twenty-four hour urine test are the preferred methods of measuring your levels of testosterone.

## DHEA

- DHEA is an androgen made by your adrenal glands, but a small amount is also made in your brain and skin.

- Women are more sensitive to the effects of DHEA than men, and therefore they need less DHEA than men do.

- DHEA has been shown to have a protective effect against cancer, diabetes, obesity, high cholesterol, heart disease, and autoimmune diseases.

## Cortisol

- Cortisol is the only hormone in your body that increases in amount with age.

- Cortisol is commonly known as the "stress hormone" due to its involvement in your response to stress. When you are stressed, cortisol levels elevate. As stress decreases, levels come back down.

- High levels of cortisol are associated with numerous symptoms and diseases, including a suppressed immune system and weight gain.

- Your adrenal glands can become "burnt out" due to over-stimulation. This is called adrenal fatigue.

• Many women enter menopause with progesterone loss due to exhaustion of their adrenal glands.

• Herbs, extracts, pregnenolone, DHEA, cortef, and stress reduction techniques are effective treatments for adrenal dysfunction.

• The simplest way to stop your cortisol levels from increasing is to better manage your stress.

## Pregnenolone

• Pregnenolone is a steroid hormone. It is a precursor to (makes) DHEA, progesterone, estrogen, testosterone, and cortisol.

• Pregnenolone makes your other sex hormones, and therefore should not be used unless you have your levels measured, since it can lead to an imbalance of your other sex hormones.

• Pregnenolone can be applied as a cream or taken by mouth.

• Pregnenolone is used for the treatment of arthritis, depression, memory loss, fatigue, and moodiness.

## Insulin

• Insulin helps regulate your blood sugar.

• If you eat too much sugar, your body produces more and more insulin until the insulin does not work as effectively as it should. This can result in high insulin levels all of the time, which can lead to your body's hormones making androgens instead of estrogens. It can also lead to insulin resistance and diabetes.

• Elevated insulin levels can be lowered by eating a balanced diet of carbohydrates, proteins, and fats. There are also nutrients that can help lower insulin levels and make insulin work better in the body.

## Thyroid Hormone

• Your thyroid gland is your body regulator. Therefore, an imbalance of your thyroid hormone can affect every metabolic function in your body.

• Since your thyroid is your body regulator, it needs to be functioning at an optimal level.

• There are a few different types of thyroid hormones that your body produces. They are:

Diiodothyronine (T2).

Thyroid Stimulating Hormone (TSH), which is made in your pituitary gland located in your brain.

Thyroxine (T4), which is made in your thyroid gland.

Triiodothyronine (T3), which is made in other tissues.

• If your thyroid is not functioning optimally, then you won't build muscle.

• Most people who are taking thyroid replacement need to take both T3 and T4.

• Nutrition and nutrients are a very important part of how well your thyroid functions.

• Medications can affect your body's ability to make thyroid hormone.

• Toxins can affect thyroid function.

• Your other hormones greatly affect how your thyroid hormone is working.

• It is important that your doctor test your entire thyroid panel and not just your TSH to see if you are hypothyroid.

• Your body needs to be able to convert T4 to T3. T3 is the more active form of thyroid hormone. This conversion requires an enzyme called 5'diodinase.

- Reverse T3 is a measurement of inactive thyroid function.

- It is very difficult to lose weight and keep it off if your reverse T3 levels remain elevated.

- If you produce too much thyroid hormone, you will get hyperthyroidism.

- Hyperthyroidism can be a life-threatening disease so it is to always be managed by your doctor.

## Melatonin

- Melatonin sets your body's twenty-four-hour cycle.

- Melatonin has an influence on many of your body's functions.

- Melatonin is an immune stimulator.

- You should have your melatonin levels measured if you have insomnia, if you have cancer, or if you are perimenopausal or menopausal.

## Prolactin

- Prolactin is made by your pituitary gland, which is located in your brain.

- Prolactin regulates nursing after childbirth. It also decreases ovarian hormone production after delivery, which helps prevent a new pregnancy while you are still nursing your baby.

# PART II: AILMENTS AND PROBLEMS

## Cervical Dysplasia

- Cervical dysplasia is the term used to describe abnormal cells on the surface of the cervix (the lowest part of the uterus).

- Cervical dysplasia doesn't cause health problems, but it is considered a pre-cancerous liaison.

- Numerous vitamin deficiencies have been associated with cervical dysplasia and cervical cancer.

- The best time to catch and begin treatment for cervical dysplasia is in the beginning stages, before the cells become cancerous. A Pap smear or colposcopy (examination of the cervix and vagina) are the best ways of discovering a problem.

## Diethylstilbestrol (DES) Babies

- Diethylstilbestrol (DES) is a synthetic, nonsteroidal estrogenic compound first made in the late 1930s.

- DES was approved for four uses: gonorrheal vaginitis (vaginal inflammation), atrophic vaginitis (which results from lower estrogen levels after menopause, causing the vaginal tissue to become drier and thinner), menopause symptoms, and postpartum lactation suppression.

- In the 1970s, it was revealed that DES had some negative side effects—for the women who took DES but mainly for the children of women who took DES while pregnant (DES babies).

- Daughters of mothers who used DES (DES daughters) have an increased risk of developing an abnormal type of vaginal cancer called adenocarcinoma, a cancer that originates in the glandular tissue. Recent studies have shown that DES can also cause abnormalities in the reproductive tract, immune system, and brain.

- Sons of mothers who took DES (DES sons) can be affected too. According to studies, DES sons are at a higher risk for epididymal cysts.

## Endometriosis

• Endometriosis is a disorder of the female reproductive system. In endometriosis, the cells that form the lining of the uterus (the endometrium) grow outside of the uterus, usually in the abdomen, pelvis, fallopian tubes, or ovaries.

• These areas of tissue growing outside the uterus are called "uterine implants." When you menstruate, the uterine implant bleeds the same way it would if it were inside your uterus; thickening, breaking down, and bleeding. This process sets up an inflammatory condition which is an irritant and causes pain, since there is nowhere for the blood to go.

• The implants produce their own estrogen by a process called "aromatization." Aromatase is an enzyme that increases the conversion of androgens (like testosterone) to estrogens in the peripheral tissues.

• If your mother or sister has endometriosis, you are more likely to have it.

• The pain you experience may not correlate with the extent of the disease. You can have large areas of endometriosis and little pain, or you can have only a few areas of endometriosis and a great deal of pain. The amount of pain seems to be determined by the depth of the lesions of endometriosis as opposed to the amount of tissue involved.

• The only definitive way to diagnose endometriosis is by laparoscopy, which is when the doctor looks inside your abdomen and takes a biopsy specimen.

## Fibrocystic Breast Disease

• Fibrocystic breast disease is a condition where there are noncancerous changes, or cysts, in the tissues of the breasts, causing pain and discomfort.

• Symptoms are at their worst before each period.

• Breast exams, mammograms, and breast examinations are effective in diagnosing fibrocystic breast disease. However, sometimes a biopsy is necessary.

• Common causes of fibrocystic breast disease are estrogen dominance, iodine deficiency, and excessive intake of caffeine.

## Fibroids

• Fibroids are benign (non-cancerous) growths on or within the walls of the uterus.

• Fibroids are a variety of sizes and quantities. Larger fibroids can cause pain, excessive bleeding, problems urinating, infertility, and premature labor.

• Certain nutrients can shrink fibroids naturally to help avoid surgery or other procedures.

• Fibroids have estrogen receptors and are thus responsive to the body's level of estrogen.

• When estrogen levels are higher, fibroids tend to grow. When estrogen levels are lower, fibroids tend to shrink.

## Heart Disease

• Heart disease is not a specific disease, but rather a broad term used to describe a number of diseases that can affect your heart and in some cases, your blood vessels.

• Heart disease is the number one killer of men and women worldwide.

• Many people think that if they watch their cholesterol, they will drastically reduce their risk of developing heart disease. However, cholesterol is only part of the picture—one-half of women who die of heart disease have normal cholesterol levels.

• Common risk factors for heart disease are age, blood pressure, diabetes, diet, gender, genetics, dental hygiene, lack of exercise, obesity, smoking, and stress.

• It is important that as a woman you have your other risk factors (besides cholesterol) of heart disease measured. The risk factors you need to look out for are homocysteine, iron (ferritin), lipoprotein A, fibrinogen, and C-reactive protein.

## Menopause

• Menopause is defined as the permanent end of menstruation and fertility.

• In the United States, 3,500 women enter menopause every day.

• Menopause occurs naturally in women when the ovaries begin making less estrogen and progesterone.

• If your hormonal symphony is out of tune, you can begin to have symptoms of menopause as early as fifteen years prior to actual menopause.

• The average age to go through menopause ranges from thirty-five to fifty-five.

• A hysterectomy (sometimes called surgical menopause) can cause menopause to occur earlier than anticipated. Even if you have had a partial hysterectomy (one or both ovaries left in) it may cause menopause to occur earlier than anticipated.

• Most women gain some weight during menopause.

• The diagnosis of menopause is made by your physician when you have had no cycle for one year and your blood levels of FSH and LH are elevated.

• The treatment you need at menopause is as individualized as your own fingerprint.

The goal is to not only alleviate symptoms but to also prevent disease.

• Surgical menopause is the removal of the ovaries in women who haven't yet experienced natural menopause. The uterus may be removed as well.

## Migraines

• Migraines are severe, painful headaches with often disabling symptoms.

• At ovulation, estrogen levels drop and progesterone levels elevate. This causes some women to get migraine headaches.

• Many women who have menstrual migraines have them due to the sudden withdrawal of progesterone that occurs just before the cycle starts. Augmenting progesterone on days twenty-two to twenty-five of the menstrual cycle will ensure that the drop in progesterone is not so abrupt. This helps many women decrease the severity and number of menstrually-related migraine headaches.

• Synthetic progesterone (progestin) in birth control pills can increase the frequency and severity of migraine headaches that are both hormonally and non-hormonally related.

## Osteoporosis

• Osteoporosis is a disease in which bones become more fragile and more likely to break. If untreated, it can progress painlessly until a bone breaks.

• The most common places people with osteoporosis experience fractures are the hip, the spine, and the wrists.

• In the United States, almost half of the women over sixty years old have osteoporosis.

- There are many risk factors for osteoporosis. One of the main ones people do not recognize is stress. Adrenal dysfunction is associated with bone loss.

- Genetics is a big risk factor for osteoporosis. Testing is available from Genova Diagnostics to see if you have this predisposition.

- To maintain your bone health, your body needs calcium, magnesium, boron, zinc, copper, silicon, phosphorus, manganese, vitamins $B_6$, $B_{12}$, D, and K, folate, and strontium. Additionally, your body has to have an optimal amount of bioflavones and amino acids to maintain and build bone.

- Milk and Tums are not the best sources of calcium intake.

- Nutrients alone are not enough to prevent osteoporosis. Estrogen, progesterone, testosterone, and DHEA levels need to be optimal to maintain and build bone.

## Perimenopause

- The time just before menopause in your life is called perimenopause. This is the time when your body begins its transition into menopause, usually starting anywhere from two to eight years before menopause and lasting up until the first year after your final period.

- You may still have menstrual cycles during perimenopause, but they might become more irregular.

## Polycystic Ovarian Syndrome (PCOS)

- Polycystic Ovarian Syndrome (PCOS) is yet another female issue that results from an imbalance of hormones. It is characterized by irregular menstrual cycles and excess testosterone production.

- Women with PCOS may have difficulties getting pregnant.

- Your chance of developing PCOS is higher if other women in your family (on your mother's or your father's side) have PCOS, irregular periods, or diabetes.

- If you are experiencing any of the symptoms associated with PCOS, it is important to see a doctor.

## Postpartum Depression

- After a pregnancy, your body resets its hormonal levels, which sometimes results in an imbalance in hormonal function. Because of this, some women experience postpartum depression.

- To tell the difference between the baby blues (a short-term, lesser degree of depression) and postpartum depression, your doctor will likely administer a depression-screening questionnaire and a few blood tests.

- Postpartum depression is not exclusive to first-time moms. It can occur after the birth of any child.

- Antidepressants, counseling, hormone replacement, and therapy are all ways to treat postpartum depression.

## Preconception Medicine

- If you are planning on conceiving, it would be beneficial to have a preconception medicine evaluation done to see what all your hormone levels are.

- Preconception medicine is a field of medicine that Metabolic/Anti-Aging physicians specialize in.

- Cigarette smoking, abuse of alcohol, and recreational drugs all affect your health and, subsequently, the health of your child.

- Stress, diet, and certain herbs can all have negative effects on pregnancy and childbirth.

## Premature Ovarian Decline (POD)

- With POD, hormone production begins to decrease at an early age. However, women with POD still have follicles in their ovaries and still experience menstrual cycles.

## Premature Ovarian Failure (POF)

- POF refers to a loss of normal hormonal function at an early age.

- POF is defined as the end of menstrual cycles before the age of thirty-five.

- Early loss of follicles in the ovaries, viruses, endocrine disruptors, autoimmune diseases, or any other disorder that prevents the ovaries from functioning normally can all cause POF.

- If POF runs in your family, your risk of developing the disease is greater.

- To diagnose POF, doctors will likely ask questions about a patient's symptoms, menstrual patterns, and history of exposure to toxins. Most sufferers show few symptoms, so a physical exam (including a pelvic exam and blood tests) is usually necessary as well.

## Premenstrual Dysphoric Disorder (PMDD)

- Premenstrual dysphoric disorder (PMDD) is a condition that is associated with severe emotional and physical symptoms that are linked to the menstrual cycle. It is considered to be a severe form of PMS.

- PMDD is distinguished from PMS by the intensity and severity of its symptoms. The symptoms of PMDD are often so severe that they are considered disabling, meaning they

get in the way of daily activities and relationships.

- The symptoms PMDD sufferers experience may change from month to month.

- In order to be diagnosed with PMDD, your symptoms must be severe enough to really disrupt your life. In other words, the symptoms interfere with work, school, relationships, and/or social activities.

- PMDD treatment is designed to minimize or eliminate symptoms.

## Premenstrual Syndrome (PMS)

- Premenstrual Syndrome (PMS) is a hormonal disorder that is characterized by the monthly recurrence of physical or psychological symptoms during the last two weeks of your cycle.

- PMS affects between 60 and 75 percent of women in the United States.

- PMS has many symptoms associated with it. Some of these symptoms affect weight gain, such as abdominal bloating, appetite changes, and salt and sugar cravings.

- Menstrual cramps are one of the most common symptoms of PMS, affecting almost 50 percent of menstruating women.

- The cause of PMS is not known, but changes in hormones during the menstrual cycle are definitely an important consideration.

- Deficiencies in certain vitamins and minerals, such as vitamin B6, calcium, and magnesium, can make the symptoms of PMS worse.

- There are many different ways to treat PMS, from medications and hormonal therapies, to nutrients and herbal modalities, to life-style changes.

- PMS can be treated with a success rate of more than 90 percent.

• Since PMS is frequently a state that is affected by low progesterone levels, progesterone supplementation has been found to be helpful.

## Skin Problems

• Your skin can be a good indicator of what is happening on the inside of your body.

• Collagen, which helps keep your skin firm and strong, requires vitamin C to be made. Therefore, if your vitamin C levels are low, your skin may age.

• Skin cells have estrogen receptors. As your estrogen levels start declining, there is a decrease in the elastin and collagen production in your connective tissue.

• Estrogen also helps your skin look younger by maintaining its firmness.

• Declining levels of testosterone, progesterone, and growth hormone also contribute to the wrinkling of your skin.

• When it comes to skin care, one size does not fit all. You deserve a personalized approach to your anti-aging skin care program.

## Vulvodynia

• Vulvodynia is the medical term for vaginal pain.

• Food may trigger an attack of vulvodynia. Foods that contain chemicals such as citric acid, salicylic acid, and oxalates may increase pain related to vulvodynia.

## PART III: HORMONE REPLACEMENT THERAPY

## What is HRT?

• There are two types of hormone replacement—one uses synthetic hormones and the other uses natural hormones.

• When it comes to hormone replacement, the word synthetic means "not the same chemical structure that your own body makes."

• If the chemical structure of the hormone matches the chemical structure of the hormone in your body, it is called "bio-identical." Hormones that are produced in a laboratory are still called natural and bio-identical if they match the chemical structure in your body. Anything else is called synthetic.

• The government-sponsored Women's Health Initiative Program halted its study on estrogen plus progestin (synthetic progesterone, or Prempro) on July 9, 2002 because it was revealed that some of the women participating in the study had an increased risk of breast cancer.

• Additional studies, such as the Heart and Estrogen/Progestin Replacement Study Follow-Up (HERS II), agree with the findings of the Women's Health Initiative Trial.

• It is estimated that one-half of women quit taking their synthetic hormone replacement therapy after one year because they are unable to tolerate the side effects.

• "Today's truth is this: There is no magic hormone or combination of hormones that can be indiscriminately used by all women. Each woman is an individual and hormonal balance must be the ultimate goal for all women."- Joseph Collins, ND

• If you are taking natural hormone replacement, it means you are using hormones that are biologically identical to, or the same chemical structure as, the ones your body makes.

• Customized natural hormonal therapy is the best way to replace hormones safely.

• The way to ensure you get the HRT you need is to use compounded hormones. With compounded hormones, your HRT therapy will be made for your own individual needs.

• Having your hormonal therapy customized at any age helps maintain the optimal hormonal symphony for your body.

• If you are considering HRT, you should make sure you thoroughly understand how all of your body's hormones work and interact with each other.

## Hormonal Testing Methods

• You should have your hormone levels measured before you begin hormone replacement therapy, no matter what age you are.

• Measuring the hormone levels throughout your body is crucial. Not doing so can result in an incorrect prescription.

• Salivary testing and a twenty-four hour urine test are the preferred methods of hormone testing for perimenopausal women, menopausal women, and women with PMS symptoms or other hormonal imbalances.

• Salivary testing gives your doctor the ability to look at your estrogen, progesterone, and testosterone levels throughout your entire monthly cycle.

• Salivary testing measures only the "free" form of the hormones.

• Twenty-four-hour urinary testing of hormonal function is also an accurate method of measuring hormone levels and hormonal function. Urine testing is able to measure the hormone level over time and, like salivary testing, evaluates the amount of free hormones. Hormone level measurement should be repeated about three months after you begin hormone replacement therapy.

• You may also have a blood test done called the SHBG test. This test measures your levels of sex hormone binding globulin (SHBG).

• Repeated measurement of your hormone levels is needed in order for your doctor to optimize your hormone replacement therapy.

## Selective Estrogen Receptor Modulators (SERMs)

• Selective estrogen receptor modulators (SERMs) are a type of hormone replacement therapy.

• Some estrogen receptor modulators, such as estriol (E3), are made inside your body. These are called endogenous estrogen receptor modulators.

• There are also exogenous estrogen receptor modulators which are made from external sources like plants (phytoestrogens) and pharmaceutical medications like tamoxifen.

• SERMs work by blocking the effects of estrogen in your breast tissue. Since SERMs are selective, as their name informs, they only block estrogen from one type of cell—the breast tissue cell.

• There are three types of SERMs: tamoxifen, raloxifene, and toremifene. They are all taken in pill form.

• Tamoxifen (brand name Nolvadex) is given to women who have had cancer to help prevent a recurrence. It works by blocking estrogen's effects on your breast tissue since it occupies the cellular receptor sites for estrogen.

• Tamoxifen does not block estrogen's affects elsewhere in your body—only on your breast tissues. Consequently, it can double or triple your risk of cancer of the uterus. It can also increase your risk of blood clots.

• Raloxifene (brand name Evista) is also a SERM. It has selective estrogen activity for bones, which means it helps maintain bone structure and therefore decreases the risk of osteoporosis.

• Raloxifene can increase bone density up to 20 percent and has been shown to decrease your risk of breast cancer.

• Toremifene (brand name Fareston) is used to treat post-menopausal women who have been diagnosed with advanced hormone-receptor-positive breast cancer.

• SERMs are not very effective in lowering triglycerides and they do not increase HDL (good cholesterol) as well as synthetic or natural hormone replacement therapies do.

• SERMs do not help maintain memory like synthetic or natural estrogens do.

## Birth Control Pills

• If you are going to take birth control pills, it is important that you supplement with a pharmaceutical-grade multivitamin to replace the nutrients that are depleted with this kind of medication.

• Estrogen-containing birth control pills decrease vitamins $B_6$, $B_{12}$, and folate in your body.

• Birth control pills can deplete your body of zinc and can elevate copper levels in your system.

• Even low-dose birth control pills contain more estrogens and progestin than the amount that is usually needed for treatment of peri-menopause or menopause.

• Birth control pills may not be the optimal HRT for perimenopausal and menopausal women.

## Nutrition and HRT

• Proper nutrition plays an important part in maximizing your HRT, preventing disease, and general treatment of menopause.

• Herbal supplements are wonderful to help resolve symptoms like hot flashes and night sweats. However, they may not be enough to maintain your bone structure, prevent heart disease, or help you maintain your memory.

• Do not use the herbal remedies in this book if you are pregnant, nursing, or if you have been diagnosed with breast cancer. All of these herbs can interfere with the efficacy of birth control pills and hormone replacement.

• Do not take black cohosh if you are taking an antidepressant.

• Chasteberry may interfere with dopamine antagonist medications.

# Resources

To find a fellowship-trained, board certified, master's prepared physician in your area who specializes in customized, prescription hormone replacement, contact the American Academy of Anti-Aging Physicians.

**American Academy of Anti-Aging Physicians**
1510 West Montana Street
Chicago, IL 60614
1-733-528-1000
www.worldhealth.net

## COMPOUNDING PHARMACIES

**Professional Compounding Centers of America**
9901 South Wilcrest Drive
Houston, TX 77099
1-800-331-2498
www.pccarx.com

## LABORATORIES

**Doctor's Data Laboratory**
3755 Illinois Avenue
St. Charles, IL 60174
1-800-323-2784
www.doctorsdata.com

**Genova Diagnostic Laboratory**
63 Zillicoa Street
Asheville, NC 28801
1-800-522-4762
www.genovadiagnostics.com

**ImmunoScience, Inc.**
325 South 3rd Street, #1-107
Las Vegas, NV 89101
1-800-522-2783
www.immunoscience.com

**Metametrix Clinical Laboratory**
3425 Corporate Way
Duluth, GA 30096
1-800-221-4640
www.metametrix.com

**NeuroScience, Inc.**
373 280th Street
Osceola, WI 54020
1-888-342-7272
www.neurorelief.com

**Spectracell Laboratories**
10401 Town Park Drive
Houston, TX 77072
1-800-227-5227
www.spectracell.com

**ZRT Laboratory**
8605 SW Creekside Place
Beaverton, OR 97006
1-503-466-2445
www.zrtlab.com

## SUPPLEMENTS

All supplements discussed in this book are available through:

**Billie Sahley, PhD**
**Pain & Stress Center Products**
5282 Medical Drive, Suite 160
San Antonio, TX 78229
1-800-669-2256
www.painstresscenter.com

**Designs For Health**
2 North Road
East Windsor, CT 06088
1-800-367-4325
www.designsforhealth.com

**Metagenics, Inc.**
P.O. Box 1729
Gig Harbor, WA 98332
1-800-843-9660
www.metagenics.com

**Ortho Molecular Products**
129 East Calhoun Street
Woodstock, IL 60098
1-815-206-6500
www.orthomolecularproducts.com

**Xymogen**
725 South Kirkman Road
Orlando, FL 32811
1-800-647-6100
www.xymogen.com

# Recommended Reading

Since my intention when writing this book was to give you an overview of the topics discussed—without getting tied up in too much medical jargon—there were a few subjects I had to hold back from elaborating on. However, should you wish to learn more about these topics, the books on this list are excellent tools. I fully recommend each one. All books are available through Amazon (www.amazon.com).

*Adrenal Fatigue* by James L. Wilson, ND, DC, PhD. This is a great book on the subject, and a must-read for anyone who has adrenal issues.

*Glycemic Index Food Guide* by Dr. Shari Lieberman. This book is a great resource if you want to read about the glycemic index.

*Heart Sense for Women* by Stephan T. Sinatra, MD. In this book, Dr. Sinatra provides an excellent discussion of risk factors for heart disease—primary and other.

*Menopause and the Mind* by Claire Warga, PhD. This is an excellent book on the subject of estrogen and its effects on your brain.

*Overcoming Thyroid Disorders* by David Brownstein, MD. This short book is a good guide on the importance of optimal levels of thyroid.

*The PCOS Protection Plan* by Colette Harris and Theresa Cheung. This book is a good action plan written *by* women with PCOS *for* women with PCOS.

*What You Must Know About Vitamins, Minerals, Herbs, & More: Choosing the Nutrients That Are Right for You* by Pamela Wartain Smith, MD, MPH. In this book, you will learn how to restore and maintain your health through the use of nutrients. Additionally, you will learn how to develop your own personalized nutritional program, whether you are trying to overcome a medical condition or simply just trying to stay healthy.

# References

## PART I: HORMONES

### ESTROGEN

Abou-Dakn, M.; Sheele, M.; Strecker, J.R. "Does breast-feeding prevent breast cancer?" *Zentralblatt fur Gynakologie*. 2003; 125: 48–52.

Ahlgrimm, M. *The HRT Solution*. 1999; New York: Avery Publishing, 2255,113.

Aldercreatz, J., et al. "Western diet and western diseases: some hormonal and biochemical mechanisms and associations." *Scand J Clin Lab Invest*. 1990; 50(suppl 201).

Alkhalaf, M.; El-Mowafy, A.; Karam, S. "Growth inhibition of MCF-7 human breast cancer cells by progesterone is associated with cell differentiation and phosphorylation of Akt protein." *Eur J Ca Prev*. 2002; 11(5): 481–488.

Aloia, J., et al. "Relationship of menopause to skeletal and muscle mass." *Am J Clin Nut*. 1991; 53: 1378–1383.

Anderson, B., et al. "Estrogen replacement therapy decreases hyperandrogenicity and improves glucose homeostasis: Plasma lipids in postmenopausal women with NIDDM." *J Clinc Endocrin*. 1997; 82(2): 638–643.

Anderson, V., et al. "Estrogen, cognition and woman's risk of Alzheimer's disease." *Am J Med*. 1997; 103(3A):11S-18S.

Arnot, B. *The Breast Cancer Prevention Diet*. 1998; New York: Little Brown and Company, 34–35, 38, 82.

Asthana, S., et al."Transdermal estrogen improves memory in women with Alzheimer's disease (abstract)." *Neurosci Abst*.1996; 22: 200.

Azcoitia, I.; Leonelli, E.; et al. "Progesterone and its derivatives dihydroprogesterone and tetrahydroprogesterone reduce myelin fiber morphological abnormalities and myelin fiber loss in the sciatic nerve of aged rats." *Neurobiology of Aging*. 2003; 24: 853–860.

Bakken, K., et al. "Hormone replacement therapy and incidence of hormone-dependent cancers in the Norwegian Women and Cancer study." *Inter Jour Cancer*. 2004; 112(1): 130–134.

Bardin, A., et al. "Loss of ER beta expression as a common step in estrogen-dependent tumor progression." *Endocr Relat Cancer*. 2004; 1193: 537–551.

Barkhem, T., et al. "Differential response of estrogen receptor alpha and receptor beta to partial estrogen agonists/antagonists." *Mol Pharmacol*.1998; 54(1): 105–112.

Barnebei, V., et al. "Plasma homocysteine in women taking hormone replacement therapy: the post menopausal estrogen/progestin interventions (PEPI) trial." *J Women's Health Gend Based Med*.1999; 8(9): 1167–1172.

Baulieu, E., et al. "Progesterone as a neuroactive neurosteroid, with special references to the effect of progesterone on myelination." *Hum Reprod*. 2000; Suppl: 1–13.

Bland, J. "Cellular communication and signal transduction." *Improving Intracellar Communication in Managing Chronic Illness*. 1999; Gig Harbor, Washington: The Function Medicine Institute, 26, 127.

Bland, J. "Inflammation and age-related diseases: The neurological, cardiovascular, and immune connection." *Nutritional Improvement of Health Outcomes-The Inflammatory Disorders.* 1997; Gig Harbor, Washington: Health Comm., Inc., 276.

Bland, J. "Introduction to neuroendocrine disorders." *Functional Medicine Approaches to Endocrine Disturbances of Aging.* 2001; Gig Harbor, Washington: The Functional Medicine Institute, 57, 62, 65, 121.

Brandes, J.L. "The influence of estrogen on migraine. Mechanisms of naringenin-induced apoptotic cascade in cancer cells: involvement of estrogen receptor alpha and bets signaling." *JAMA.* 2006; 295(15): 1824–1830.

Brineat, M., et al. "Long-tern effects of the menopause and sex hormones on skin thickness." *Br J Obstet Gynaecol.* 1985; 92(3): 256–259.

Bruce, A., et al. "Estrogen attenuates and corticosterone exacerbates excitotoxin oxidative injury and amyloid beta-peptide toxicity in hippocampal neuron." *Jour of Neurochem.* 1996; 66(5): 1836–1844.

Bush, T., et al. "Preserving cardiovascular benefits of hormone replacement therapy." *Journal of Reproductive Med.* 2000; 45(3suppl): 259–273.

Canonico, M.; Oger, E.; Conard, J.; Meyers, G.; et al. "Obesity and risk of venous thromboembolism among postmenopausal women: differential impact of hormone therapy by route of estorgen administration. The ESTHER study." *J of Thromb and Haemost.* 2006; 4(6): 1259–1265.

Chadhurz, N., et al. "Antioxidant and pro-oxidant actions of estrogens: potential physiological and clinical implications." *Seminars in Reproductive Endocrin.* 1998; 16(4): 309–314.

Chetkowski, R., et al. "Biologic effects of transdermal estradiol." *NEJM.* 1986; 314: 1615–1620.

Clarkson, R. "Progesterone and cardiovascular disease. A critical review." *Jour Repro Med.* 1999; 44(2 Suppl): 180–184.

Cohen, L.S.; Soares, C.N.; Poitras, J.R.; et al. "Short-term use of estradiol for depression in perimenopausal and postmenopausal women: A preliminary report." *Am J Psychiatry.* 2003; 160: 1519–1522.

Col, N.F.; Pauker, S.G. "The discrepancy between observational studies and randomized trials of menopausal hormone therapy: did expectations shape experience?" *Ann Intern Med.* 2003; 139: 923–929.

Colacurci, N., et al. "Effects of hormone replacement therapy on glucose metabolism." *Panminerva Med.* 1998; 40(1): 18–21.

Cole, P., et al. "Oestrogen fractions during early reproductive life in the aetiology of breast cancer." *Lancet.* 1969; 1(7595): 604–606.

Collaborative Group on Hormonal Factors in Breast Cancer. "Breast cancer and breastfeeding: collaborative reanalysis of individual data from 47 epidemiological studies in 30 countries, including 50302 women with breast cancer and 96973 women without the disease." *Lancet.* 2002; 360: 187–195.

Collins, J. *What's Your Menopause Type.* 2000; Roseville, CA: Prima Health, 69.

Compton, J., et al. "HRT and its effect on normal ageing of the brain and dementia." *Brit Jour Clin Pharmacol.* 2001; 52(6): 647–653.

Crook, D. "The metabolic consequences of treating postmenopausal women with nonoral hormone replacement therapy." *Brit Jour Obstet Gynaecol.* 1997; 104(Suppl 16): 4–13.

Crook, T. *The Memory Cure.* 1998; New York: Pocket Books, p. 159.

Dalton, K. *The Premenstrual Syndrome and Progesterone Therapy.* 1984; Chicago, Illinois: Year Book Medical Publishers, Inc.

DeLellis, K.; Ingles, S.; et al. "IGF-1 genotype, mean plasma level and breast cancer risk in the Hawaii/Los Angeles multiethnic cohort." *Br J Cancer.* 2003; 88: 227–282.

Di Paolo, T., et al. "Modulation of brain dopamine transmission by sex steroids." *Rev Neurosci.* 2005; 5: 27–41.

Dimitrakakis, C.; Jones, R.; Liu, A.; Bondy, C. "Breast cancer incidene in postmenopausal women using testosterone in addition to usual hormone therapy." *Menopause.* 2004; 11: 531–535.

Drake, E., et al. "Associations between circulating sex steroid hormones and cognition in normal elderly women." *Neurology.* 2000; 54(3): 599–603.

Drew, P.D.; Chavis, J.A. "Female sex steroids; effects upon microglial cell activation." *J of Neuroimmunology.* 2000; 111(1–2): 77–85.

Drouva, S., et al. "Estradiol activates methylating enzyme(s) involved in the conversion of phosphatidyl-ethanolamine to phosphatidlyl-choline in rat pituitary membranes." *Endocrinol.* 1986; (1996): 2611–2622.

Duka, T., et al. "The effects of 3-week estrogen hormone replacement on cognition in elderly healthy females." *Psychopharmacol.* 2000; 149(2): 129–139.

Duff, S., et al. "A beneficial effect of estrogen on working memory in postmenopausal women taking hormone replacement therapy." *Horm Behav.* 2000; 38(4): 262–376.

Erenus, M., et al. "Comparison of effects of continuous combined transdermal with oral estrogen and oral progestogen replacement therapies on serum lipoproteins and compliance." *Climacteric.* 2001; 4: 228–234.

Felson, D.; Cummings, S. "Aromatase inhibitors and the syndrome of arthralgias with estrogen deprivation." *Arthritis & Rheumatism.* 2005; 52: 2594–2598.

Fink, G., et al. "Estrogen control of central neurotransmission: effect on mood, mental state, and memory." *Cellular & Mol Neurobiol.* 1996; 16(3): 325–344.

Fishman, J., et al. "Increased estrogen 16-alpha hydroxylase activity in women with breast and endometrial cancer." *J Steroid Biochem.* 1984; 20: 1077–1081.

Follingstad, A. "Estriol, the forgotten estrogen?" *JAMA.* 1978; 239(1): 29–30.

Fonseea, E., et al. "Increased serum levels of growth hormone and insulin-like growth factor(associated with simultaneous decrease of circulating insulin in postmenopausal women receiving hormone replacement therapy." *Menoapuse J North Amer Men Soc.* 1999; 61: 56–60.

Fotsis, T.; Zhang, Y.; Pepper, M.; et al. "The endogenous oestrogen metabolite 2-methoxy-oestradiol inhibits angiogenesis and suppresses tumor growth." *Nature.* 1994; 268: 237–239.

Fournier, A.; Berrino, F.; Riboi, E.; et al. "Breast cancer risk in relation to different types of hormone replacement therapy in the E3N-EPIC cohort." *International Union Against Cancer.* 2005; 114: 448–454.

Franke, H.R.; Vermes, I. "Differential effects of progestogens on breast cancer cell lines." *Maturitas.* 2003; 46(Suppl 1): S55–S58.

Gilson, G., et al. "A perspective on HRT for women: Picking up the pieces after the Women's Health Initiative Trial, Part 1." 2003; *Intern Jour of Pharmaceutical Compounding.* 7(4): 250–56, 277, 285, 291.

Giuliani, A.; Concin, H.; Wieser, F.; et al. "Hormone replacement therapy with a transdermal estradiol gel and oral micronized progesterone. Effect on menopausal symptoms and lipid metabolism." *Wien Klin Wochenschr.* 2000; 112(14): 629–633.

Greenblatt, R., et al. "The fate of a large bolus of exogenous estrogen administered to postmenopausal women." *Maturitas.* 1979; 2: 29–35.

Greendale, G., et al. "The menoapuse transition." *Endocrinol Metab Clin NA.* 1997; 26(2): 261–277.

Gross, J., et al. "Relationship between steroid excretion patterns and breast cancer incidence in Israeli women of various origins." *Jour Nat Cancer Inst.* 1997; 59(1): 7–11.

Guicheney, P., et al. "Platelet serotonin content and plasma tryptophan in peri and postmenopausal women: Variations within plasma oestrogen levels and depressive symptoms." *Euro Clinic Invest.* 1988; 18: 297–304.

Halbreich, U., et al. *CNS Drugs.* 2001; 15(10): 797–817.

Halbreich, U., et al. "Role of estrogen in postmenopausal depression." *Neurol.* 1997; 48(5): 516(Suppl 7).

Hanaway, P. "Hormone essentials: Personalizing diagnosis and treatment." Module I, Anti-Aging and Regenerative Medicine Fellowship; Las Vegas, NV; Dec. 10–12, 2007.

Hargrove, J.T.; Maxson, W.S.; Wentz, A.C.; Burnett, L.S. "Menopausal hormone replacement therapy with continuous daily oral micronized estradiol and progesterone." *Obstet Gynecol.* 1989; 73(4): 606–612.

Hays, B. "Estrogen and depression." *Disorders of the Brain: Emerging Therapies in Complex Neurologic and Psychiatric Conditions.* 2002; Gig Harbor, Washington: Institute For Functional Medicine, Inc., 269–270, 280.

Hays, B. "Solving the hormone replacement dilemma in perimenopause." *Functional Medicine Approaches To Endocrine Disturbances Of Aging*. Gig Harbor, Washington: The Institute For Function Medicine, Inc.; 2001, 15–43.

Head, K. "Estriol: Safety and efficacy." *Altern Med Rev*. 1998; 3: 101–113.

Heikkinen, A., et al. "Postmenopausal hormone replacement therapy and autoantibodies against oxidized LDL." *Maturitas*. 1998; 29(2): 155–161.

Henderson, V., et al. "Cognitive skills associated with estrogen replacement in women with Alzheimer's disease." *Psychoneuroendocrinol*. 1996; 21(4): 421–430.

Henderson, V., et al. "The epidemiology of estrogen replacement therapy and Alzheimer's disease." *Neurology*. 1997; 48: S27–S35.

Henderson, V., et al. "Estrogen replacement therapy in older women. Comparisons between Alzheimer's disease cases and nondemented control subjects." *Archieves of Neurology*. 1994; 51(9): 896–900.

Hermsmeyer, R.I.K.; Mishra, R.G.; Pavcnik, D.; Uchida, B. "Prevention of coronary hyperactivity in preatherogenic menopausal rhesus monkeys by transdermal progesterone." *Arterioscler Thromb Vasc Biol*. 2004; 24: 955–961.

Holtorf, K. "The bio-identical hormone debate: are bio-identical hormones (estradiol, estriol, and progesterone) safer or more efficient than commonly used synthetic versions in hormone replacement therapy?" *Post Grad Med*. 2009; 121(1): 1–13. http://mail.google.com/mail/images/cleardot.gif

Inukai, T., et al. "Estrogen markedly increases LDL-receptor activity in hypercholesterolemic patients." *Jour Med*. 2000; 32: 247–261.

Itoi, H., et al. "Comparison of the long-term effects of oral estriol with the effects of conjugated estrogen on serum lipid profile in early menopausal women." *Maturitas*. 2000; 36: 217–222.

Jacobs, D., et al. "Cognitive function in nondeminated older women who took estrogen after menopause." *Neurology*. 1998; 50(2): 368–373.

Jernstrom, H.; Lubinski, J.; Lynch, H.T.; et al. "Breast-feeding and the risk of breast cancer in BRCA1 and BRCA2 mutation carriers." *J Nation Ca Institute*. 2004; 96: 1094–1098.

Jezova, D., et al. "Reduction of rise in blood pressure and cortisol release during stress by Ginkgo biloba extract (EGb 761) in healthy volunteers." *Jour Physiol Pharmacol*. 2002; 53(3): 337–348.

Kampen, D., et al. "Estrogen use and verbal memory in healthy post-menopausal women." *Obstet Gynecol*. 1994; 83(6): 979–983.

Kassirer, J.P. "Why should we swallow what these studies say?" *Advanced Studies in Medicine*. 2004; 4(8): 397–398.

Kimura, D., et al. "Estrogen replacement therapy may protect against intellectual decline in postmenopausal woman." *Hormones and Behavior*. 1995; 29: 312–321.

Klaiber, E., et al. "Estrogen therapy for severe persistent depressions in women." *Arch Gen Psy*. 1979; 36: 559–554.

Koh, K., et al. "Effects of hormone replacement therapy on fibrinolysis in postmenopausal women." *NEJM*. 1997; 336: 683–690.

Koloszar, S.; Kovacs, L. "Treatment of climacteric urogenital disorders with an estiol-containing ointment." *Orv Hetil*. 1995; 136(7): 343–345.

Lauritzen, C., et al. "Results of a 5 years prospective study of estriol succinate treatment in patients with climacteric complaints." *Horm Metabol Res*. 1987; 19: 579–584.

Laux, M. *Natural Woman, Natural Menopause*. 1997; New York: HarperCollins, 20–21, 79.

Lee, J. *What Your Doctor May Not Tell You About Premenopause*. 1999; New York: Warner Books, 4.

Lemon, H., et al. "Estriol prevention of mammary carcinoma induced by 7, 12-dimethyl-benzanthracene and procarbazine." *Cancer Res*. 1975; 35: 1341–1352.

Lemon, H., et al. "Pathophysiologic considerations in the treatment of menopausal symptoms with estrogens: the role of estriol in the prevention of mammary carcinoma." *ACTA Endocrinol*. 1980; 233(suppl): 17–27.

Lemon, H., et al. "Reduced estriol excretion in patients with breast cancer prior to endocrine therapy." *JAMA*. 1966; 196(13): 1129–1136.

Liune, V., et al. "Immuno-chemical demonstration of increased choline acetyltranferase concentration in rat preoptic area after estradiol administration." *Brain Res.* 1980; 191(1): 273–277.

Lopez-Jaramillo, P., et al. "Improvement in functions of the central nervous system by estrogen replacement therapy might be related with an increased nitric oxide production." *Endothelium.* 1999; 6(4): 263–266.

Mabjeesh, N.; Escuin, D.; Lavallee, T.; Pribluda, V.; et al. "2ME2 inhibits tumor growth and angiogenesis by disrupting microtubules and dysregulating HIF." *Cancer Cell.* 2003; 3: 363–375.

MacMahon, B., et al. "Oestrogen profiles of Asian and North American women." *Lancet.* 1971; 2(7730): 900–1002.

Manonai, J., et al. "Effect of oral estriol on urogenital symptoms, vaginal cytology, and plasma hormone level in postmenopausal women." *Jour Med Assoc Thai.* 2001; 84: 539–544.

McEwen, B., et al. "Observations in a preliminary open trial of estradiol therapy for senile dementia-Alzheimer's type." *Psychneuroendocrinol.* 1986; 11(3): 337–45.

McEwen, B., et al. "Steroid and thyroid hormones modulate a changing brain." *Journal of Steroid Biochemistry and Molecular Biology.* 1991; 40(1–3): 1–14.

Melamed, M., et al. "Molecular and kinetic basis for the mixed agonist/antagonist activity of estriol." *Mol Endocrinol.* 1997; 11: 1868–1878.

Michnovicz J., et al. "Environmental modulation of oestrogen metabolism in humans." *Int'l Clin Nutr Rev.* 1987; 7(4): 169–173.

Missmer, S.A.; Eliassen, A.H.; Barbieri, R.L.; et al. "Endogenous estrogen, androgen, and progesterone concentrations and breast cancer risk among postmenopausal women." *J of the National Cancer Institute.* 2004; 96(24): 1856–1865.

Molloy, E.J.; O'Neill, A.J.; et al. "Sex-specific alterations in neutrophil spoptosis: the role of estradiol and progesterone." *Blood.* 2003; 102(7): 2653–9.

Morrison, A., et al. "A prospective study of ERT and the risk of developing Alzheimer's disease in the Baltimore longitudinal study of aging." (abstract) *Neurol.* 1996; 46: A435–A436.

Morrison, J., et al. "Life and death of neurons in the aging brain." *Science.* 1997; 278: 412–419.

Mulnard, R., et al. "Estrogen replacement therapy for treatment of mild to moderate Alzheimer's disease." *JAMA.* 2000; 283: 1007–1015.

Nabulsi, A., et al. "Association of hormone replacement therapy with various cardiovascular risk factors in post menopausal women." *NEJM.* 1993; 328: 1069–1075.

Nachtigall, L. *Estrogen The Facts Can Change Your Life.* 1995; New York: HarperCollins, 27, 33.

Nachtigall, L., et al. "Serum estradiol-binding profiles in postmenopausal women undergoing three common estrogen replacement therapies: Associations with sex hormone-binding globulin, estradiol, estrone levels." *Menopause.* 2000; 7: 243–250.

Nike, E., et al. "Estrogens as antioxidants." *Methods Enczymol.* 1990; 186: 330.

Paganini-Hill, A., et al. "Alzheimer's disease in women." *The Female Patient.* 1998; 23: 10–20.

Paganini-Hill, A., et al. "Does estrogen replacement therapy protect against Alzheimer's disease?" *Osteoporosis Int.* 1997; Suppl 1: S12–S17.

Paganini-Hill, A., et al. "Estrogen deficiency and risk of Alzheimer's disease in women." *Am J. Epidemiol.* 1994; 140: 256–261.

Paganini-Hill, A., et al. "Estrogen replacement therapy and risk of Alzheimer's disease." *Arch Intern Med.* 1996; 156: 2213–2217.

Pansini, F., et al. "Control of carbohydrate metabolism in menopausal women receiving transdermal estrogen therapy." *Ann NY Acad Sci.* 1990; 592: 460–462.

Parashar, S.; Rumsfeld, J.S.; et al. "Women, depression, and outcome of myocardial infarction." *Circulation.* 2007; 115(8).

Pasqualini, J. "The fetus, pregnancy, and breast cancer." *Breast Cancer: Prognosis, Treatment, and Prevention.* 2002; NY: Marcel Dekker Inc., 19–71.

Pawlak, K.J.; Zhang, G.; Wiebe, J.P. "Membrane 5–pregane-3, 20-dione receptors in MCR-7 and MCF-10A breast cancer cells are up-regulated by estradiol and 5 P and down regulated by the progesterone metabolites, 3-dihydroprogesterone and 20-dihydroprogesterone, with associated changes in cell proliferation and detachment." *SBMB.* 2005; 1–11.

Phillips, S., et al. "Effects of estrogen on memory function in surgically menopausal women." *Psycho Neuroendocrinology.* 1992; 17(5): 485–495.

Poehlman, E., et al. "Changes in energy balance and body composition at menopause: A controlled longitudinal study." *Ann of Int Med.* 1995; 123(9): 673–675.

Polanczyk, M.J.; Carson, B.D.; Subramanian, S.; et al. "Cutting edge : Estrogen drives expansion of the CD4+CD25+ regulatory T cell compartment." *The Journal of Immunology.* 2004; 173: 2227–2230.

Polanczyk, M.; Hopke, C.; Huan, J.; et al. "Enhanced FoxP3 expression and Treg cell function in pregnant and estrogen-treated mice." *J of Neuroimmunology.* 2005; 170(1): 85–92.

Puder, J., et al. "Estrogen modulates the hypothalamic-pituitary-adrenal and inflammatory cytokine responses to endotoxin in women." *Jour Clin Endocrinol Metab.* 2001; 86(6): 2403– 2408.

Raz, R., et al. "A controlled trial of intravaginal estriol in postmenopausal women with recurrent urinary tract infections." *NEJM.* 1993; 329: 753–756.

Rea, M.F. "Benefits of breastfeeding and women's health." *Jornal de Pediatria.* 2004; 80: S142–S146.

Reed, M.J.; Purohit, A. "Breast cancer and the role of cytokines in regulating estrogen synthesis: an emerging hypothesis." *Endocrine Reviews.* 1997; 18(5): 701–715.

Reichman, M., et al. "Effects of alcohol consumption on plasma and urinary hormone concentrations in premenopausal women." *Jour Nat Cancer Inst.* 1993; 85(9): 692–693.

Rice, M., et al. "Estrogen replacement therapy and cognitive function in postmenopausal women without dementia." *Am J Med.* 1997; 103(3A): 26S-35S.

Rich, R., et al. "Kinetic analysis of estrogen receptor/ligand interactions." *Proc Nat Acad Sci USA.* 2002; 99(13): 8562–8567.

Richer, J.K.; Lange, C.A.; Manning, N.G.; et al. "Convergence of progesterone with growth factor and cytokine signaling in breast cancer. Progesterone receptors regulate signal transducers and activators of transcription expression and activity." *J of Biol Chem.* 1998; 273(47): 31317–31326.

Richman, S.; Edusa, V.; Ahmed, F.; et al. "Low-dose estrogen therapy for prevention of osteoporosis: working our way back to monotherapy." *Menopause.* 2006; 13(1): 148–155.

Rosano, G., et al. "Syndrome X in women is associated with estrogen deficiency." *Eur Heart J.* 1995; 16:610: 14.

Rosner, B., et al. "Reproductive risk factors in a prospective study of breast cancer: the Nurses' Health study." *Amer Jour Epidemiol.* 1994; 139(8): 819–835.

Rouzier, N. "Estrogen and progesterone replacement." *Longevity and Preventive Medicine Symposium.* 2002; 8.

Russo, J., et al., "Differentiation of the mammary gland and susceptibility to carcinogenesis," *Breast Cancer Res Treat.* 1982; 2(1):5–73.

Santaro, N.; Rosenberg-Brown, J.; et al. "Characterization of reproductive hormonal dynamics in the perimenopause." *J Clin Endo Metab.* 1996; 81: 1495–1501.

Sarrel, P., et al. "Estrogen actions in arteries, bone and brain." *Sci Am Med.* 1994; 1: 44.

Sarrel, P., et al. "Ovarian hormones: recent findings of cardiological significance." *Cardiology in Practice.* 1991; Mar-Apr 14–17.

Scarabin, P., et al. "Effects of oral and transdermal estrogen/progesterone regimens on blood coagulation and fibrinolysis in postmenopausal women," A randomized controlled trial." *Arterioscler Thromb Vasc Biol.* 1997; 17: 3071–3078.

Seely, E.W.; Walsh, B.W.; Gerhard, M.D.; Williams, G.H. "Estradiol with or without progesterone and ambulatory blood pressure in postmenopausal women." *Hypertension.* 1999; 33(5): 1190–1194.

Sephton, S.E.; Sapolsky, R.M.; Kraemer, H.C.; et al. "Diurnal cortisol rhythm as a predictor of breast cancer survival." *J Natl Cancer Inst.* 2000; 92(12): 994–1000.

Shaywitz, S., et al. "Effect of estrogen on brain activation patterns in postmenopausal women during working memory tasks." *JAMA.* 1999; 281(13): 1197–2002.

Sherman, B., et al. "Estrogen use and verbal memory in healthy postmenopausal women." *Obstet and Gynecol.* 1994; 83(6): 979–983.

Sherwin, B., et al. "Estrogen and cognitive functioning in surgically menopausal women." *Ann NY Acad Sci.* 1990; 592: 474–475.

Sherwin, B., et al. "Estrogen effects on cognition in menopausal women." *Neurology.* 1997: 48(Suppl 7): S21–S26.

Sherwin, B., et al. "Estrogen use and verbal memory in healthy post-menopausal women." *Obstetrics & Gyn.* 1994; 83(6): 979–983.

Singletary, K., et al. "Alcohol and breast cancer: review of epidemiologic and experimental evidence and potential mechanisms." *JAMA.* 2001; 286: 2143–2151.

Shippen, E. *Testosterone Syndrome.* 1998; New York: M. Evans & Company Inc., 145.

Short, R.V. "What the breast does for the baby, and what the baby does for the breast." *Australian and New Zealand Journal of Obste and Gyne.* 1994; 34: 262–264.

Simpkins, J., et al. "Estrogen and memory protection." *Jour Soc of Obstet & Gyn of Canada.* 1997; (Suppl): 14–16.

Simpkins, J., et al. "Estrogen may be useful therapy for Alzheimer's disease and other neurodegenerative diseases." *Am J. Med.* 1997; 103(3A): 19S-23S.

Sinatra, S. *Heart Sense for Women.* 2000; Washington D.C.: LifeLine Press, 108, 164, 205, 206, 207, 208, 210, 211.

Sinatra, S. *Optimum Health.* 1996; Gatlinburg, TN: The Lincoln-Bradley Publishing Group; p. 164.

Smigel, K.L. "Breast-feeding linked to decreased cancer risk for mother, child."

*J of the Nation Ca Inst.* 1988; 80(17): 1362–1363.

Sonni, R.; Bondi, G.; Travaglini, S. "Presenile and senile vulvovaginitis. Topical hormonal treatment with estriol." *Minerva Ginecol.* 1991; 43(4): 177–179.

Speroff, L. "The breast as an endocrine target organ." *Contemp Obstet Gynec.* 1977; 9: 69–72.

Stamm, W., et al. "A controlled trial of intravaginal estriol in postmenopausal women with urinary tract infections." *NEJM.* 1993; 329(11): 753–756.

Stevens, M., et al. "Low-dose estradiol alters brain activity." *Psychiatry Res.* 2005; 139(3): 199–217.

Strivastava, R., et al. "Apoliporpotein E gene expression in various tissues of mouse and regulation by estrogen." *Biochem Mol Biol Int.* 1996; 38: 91–101.

Studd, J., et al. "Hormones and depression in women." *Climacteric.* 2004; 7(4): 338–46.

Sudhir, L., et al. "Estrogen supplementation decreases norepinephrine-induced vasoconstriction and total body norepinephrine spillover in perimenopausal women." *Hypertension.* 1997; 30(6):1538–1543.

Takahashi, K., et al. "Safety and efficacy of oestriol for symptoms of natural or surgically induced menopause." *Hum Repro.* 2000; 15: 1028–1036.

Tang, M., et al. "Effect of oestrogen during menopause on risk and age at onset of Alzheimer's disease." *Lancet.* 1996; 348: 429–432.

Taylor, M. "Unconventional estrogens: Estriol, biest, and triest." *Clin Obstet Gynecol.* 2001; 44: 864–879.

*The Importance of Detoxification.* 2002; Advanced Nutritional Publications, Inc.

Thompson, N., et al. "Exisulind induction of apoptosis involves guanosine 3,5-cyclic monophosphate phosphodiesterase inhibitor, protein kinase activation and attenuated B-catenin." *Cancer Res.* 2000; 60: 3338–3342.

Totta, P.; Acconcia, F.; Leone, S.; et al. "Mechanisms of naringenin-induced apoptotic cascade in cancer cells: involvement of estrogen receptor alpha and beta signaling." *IUBMB Life.* 2004 Aug: 56(8): 491–9.

Turner-Cobb, J.M.; Sephton, S.E.; Koopman, C.,; et al. "Social support and salivary cortisol in women with metastatic breast cancer." *Psychosom Med.* 2000; 62(3): 337–345.

Tzay-Shing, Y., et al. "Efficacy and safety of estriol replacement therapy for climacteric women." *Chin Med J.* (Taipei) 1995; 55: 386–391.

Tzingourius, V., et al. "Estriol in the management of the menopause." *JAMA.* 1978; 239: 1638–1641.

Ursin, G., et al. "Do urinary estrogen metabolites reflect the differences in breast cancer risk between Singapore Chinese and United States African-American and white women?" *Cancer Res.* 2001; 61(8): 3326–3329.

Ushiroyama, T., et al. "Estrogen replacement therapy in postmenopausal women: A study of the efficacy of estriol and changes in plasma gonadotropin levels." *Gynecol Endocrinol.* 2001; 15: 74–80.

Van Baal, W., et al. "Cardiovascular disease risk and hormone replacement therapy(HRT). A review based on randomized, controlled studies in postmenopausal women." *Curr Med Chem.* 2000; 7(5): 499–517.

Van der Linden, M., et al. "The effect of estriol on the cytology of urethra and vagina in postmenopausal women with genito-urinary symptoms." *Eur J Obstet Gynecol Reprod Biol.* 1993; 51(1): 29–33.

Van den Heuvel, M.W.; Van Bragt, A.J.; et al. "Comparison of ethinylestradiol pharmacokinetics in three hormonal contraceptive formulations: the vaginal ring, the transdermal patch, and an OC." *Contraception.* 2005; 72: 168–174.

Vatten, L., et al. "Pregnancy related protection against breast cancer depends on length of gestation." *Brit Jour Cancer.* 2002; 87(3): 289–90.

Vehkavaara, S., et al. "Effects of oral and transdermal estrogen replacement therapy on markers of coagulation, fibrinolysis, inflammation and serum lipids and lipoproteins in postmenopausal women." *Throm Haemost.* 2001; 85: 619–625.

Vliet, E., et al. "New insights on hormones and mood." *Menopause Management.* 1993; June/July: 140–146, 203, 217–218, 224, 302.

Vliet, E. *Women Weight and Hormones.* 2001; New York: M. Evans & Company, 25, 39, 45, 69, 81, 84–85, 88, 99–100, 140, 145.

Vongpatanasin, W., et al. "Transdermal estrogen replacement therapy decreases sympathetic activity in postmenopausal women." *Circulation.* 2001; 103: 2903–2908.

Warga, C. *Menopause and the Mind.* 1999; New York: Simon and Schuster, XVII, 92, 284.

Weiland, N. "Estradiol selectively regulates against binding sites on the N-Methyl-D-Aspartate receptor complex in the CA1 region of the hippocampus." *Endocrinology.* 1992; 131: 662–668.

Whitley, B.R.; Palmieri, D., Twerdi, C.D.; et al. "Expression of active plasminogen activator inhibitor-1 reduces cell migration and invasion in breast and gynecological cancer cells." *Exp Cell Res.* 2004; 296(2): 151–162.

Whooley, M.; McCaffery, J.; et al. "Association of serotonin transporter polymorphism (5–HTTLPR) with depression, perceived stress, and norepinephrine in patients with coronary disease: The Heart and Soul Study." *Circulation.* 2007; 115(8).

Williams, G., et al. "Modulation of memory fields by dopamine D1 receptors in prefrontal cortex." *Nature.* 1995; 376(6541): 572–575.

Wise, P., et al. "Minireview: neuroprotective effects of estrogen—new insights in mechanisms of action." *Endocrinol.* 2001; 142(3): 969–973.

Xu, H., et al. "Estrogen reduces neuronal generation of Alzheimer's B-amyloid peptides." *Nature Med.* 1998; 4(4): 447–451.

Yaffe, K., et al. "Apolipoprotein E phenotype and cognitive decline in a prospective study of elderly community women." *Arch Neuro.* 1998; 54: 1110–1114.

Yaffe, K., et al. "Cognitive decline in women in relation to non-protein-bound oestradiol concentrations." *Lancet.* 2000; 356: 708–712.

Yaffe, K., et al. "Estrogen therapy in postmenopausal women: effects on cognitive function and dementia." *JAMA.* 1998; 279(9): 688–695.

Yang, T.S.; Tsan, S.H.; Chang, S.P.; Ng, H.T. "Efficacy and safety of estriol replacement therapy for climacteric women." *Zhonghua Yi Xue Za Zhi (Taipei).* 1995; 55(5): 386–391.

Yu, H.; Shu, X.O.; et al. "Plasma sex steroid hormones and breast cancer risk in Chinese women." *Inter J Ca.* 2003; 105(1): 92–97.

Yue, T.; Wang, X.; Louden, C.S.; et al. "2-Methoxyestradiol, and endogenous estrogen metabolite, induces apoptosis in endothelial cells and inhibits angiogenesis : Possible role for stress-activated protein kinase signaling pathway and Fas expression." *Molecular Pharmacology.* 1997; 51: 951–962.

Zandi, P., et al. "Hormone replacement therapy and incidence of Alzheimer disease in older women." *JAMA.* 2002; 288(17): 2123–2129.

Zhu, B., et al. "Quantitative structure-activity relationship of various endogenous estrogen metabolites for human estrogen receptor alpha and beta subtypes: insights into the structural determinants favoring a differential subtype binding." *Endocrinol.* 2006; 147(9): 4132–4150.

## PROGESTERONE

Adams, M., et al. "Medroxyprogesterone acetate antagonized inhibitory effects of conjugated equine estrogens on coronary artery atherosclerosis." *Arterioscler Thromb Vasc Biol.* 1997; 17: 217–221.

Anasti, J.N.; Leonetti, H.B.; Wilson, K.J. "Topical progesterone cream has antiproliferative effect on estrogen-stimulated endometrium." *Obstet Gynecol.* 2001; 97: S10.

Azcoitia, I.; Leonelli, E.; et al. "Progesterone and its derivatives dihydroprogesterone and tetrahydroprogesterone reduce myelin fiber morphological abnormalities and myelin fiber loss in teh sciatic nerve of aged rats." *Neurobiology of Aging.* 2003; 24(6): 853–860.

Backstom, T. "Epileptic seizures in women related to plasma estrogen and progesterone during the menstrual cycle." *Acta Neurol Scand.* 1976 Oct. 54(4): 321–347.

Baghurst, P., et al. "Diet, prolactin and breast cancer." *Am J Clin Nutr.* 1992; 56: 943–949.

Bender, S. *The Power of Perimenopause.* 1998; New York: Harmony Books, p. 168.

Bergerson, R.; Demontigny, C.; Debonnel, G. "Potentiation of neuronal NMDA response induced by dehydroepiandrosterone and its suppression by progesterone: effects mediated via sigma receptors." *The Journal of Neuroscience.* 1996; 16(3): 1193–1202.

Beynon, H.L.; Garbett, N.D.; Banres, P.J. "Severe premenstrual exacerbations of asthma: effect of intramuscular progesterone." *Lancet.* 1988 Aug. 13; 2(8607): 370–2.

Bland, J. "Introduction to neuroendocrine disorders." *Functional Medicine Approaches to Endocrine Disturbances of Aging.* 2001; Gig Harbor, Washington: The Functional Medicine Institute, 57, 65–66.

Brady, B.M.; Anderson, R.A.; et al. "Demonstration of progesterone receptor-mediated gonadotrophin suppression in the human mal." *Clin Endo.* 2003; 58(4): 506–12.

Brownstein, D. *Overcoming Thyroid Disorders.* 2002; West Bloomfield, MI: Medical Alternatives Press, 8, 113.

Bumke-Bogt, C.; Bahr, V.; Diederich, S.; et al. "Expression of the progesterone receptor and progesterone-metabolizing enzymes in the female and male human kidney." *J of Endocrin.* 2002; 175(2): 349–64.

Burry, K.; Patton, P.; Hermsmeyer, K. "Percutaneous absorption of progesterone in postmenopausal women treated with transdermal estrogen." *American Journal of Obstetric Gynecology.* 1999; 180: 1504–1511.

Campagnoli, C., et al. "Progestins and progesterone in hormone replacement therapy and the risk of breast cancer." *Jour Steroid Biochem Mol Biol.* 2005; 96(2): 95–108.

Cermody, B.J.; Arora, S.; et al. "Progesterone inhibits human infragenicular arterial smooth muscle cell proliferation induced by high glucose and insulin concentrations." *J Vasc Surg.* 2002; 36: 833–8.

Choi, B.C.; Polgar, K.; et al. "Progesterone inhibits in-vitro embryotoxic Th1 cytokine production to trophoblast in women with recurrent pregnancy loss." *Human Reproduction.* 2000. 15 Suppl 1: 46–59.

Clarkson, T., et al. "Conjugated equine estrogens alone, but not in combination with medroxyprogesterone acetate, inhibit aortic connective tissue remodeling after plasma lipid lowering in female monkeys." *Arterioscler Thromb Vasc Biol.* 1998; 18(7): 1164–1171.

Colditz, G., et al. "Use of estrogen plus progestin is associated with greater increase in brest cancer risk than estrogen alone." *Am J. Epidemiol.* 1998; 147(suppl): 64S.

Collins, J. *What's Your Menopause Type.* 2000; Roseville, CA: Prima Health, 67.

Dalton, K. *The Premenstrual Syndrome and Progesterone Therapy 2nd ed.* 1984; London, England; Chicago, Ill: Year Book Medical Publishers.

DeMasi, M. "Hormonally associated migrane." *The Female Patient.* 2004; 29(7): 30–36.

Donghai, et al. "Progesterone inhibits human endometrial cancer cell growth and invasiveness: downregulation of cellular adhesion molecules through progesterone B receptors." *Cancer Research.* 2002; 62: 881–886.

"Drugs that cause sexual dysfuction: an update." *The Medical Letter.* 1992; 34 (Issue 876).

Dzugan, S, et al. "Progesterone misconceptions." *Life Extension.* April 2006; p. 49–55.

Dzugan, S., et al. "The simultaneous restoration of neurohormonal and metabolic integrity as a very promising method of migraine management." *Bull Urg Rec Med.* 2003; 4(4): 62–68.

Ferrell, R.; O'Connor, K.; Rodririguez, G.; et al. "Monitoring reproductive aging in a 5-year prospective study: aggregate and individual changes in steroid hormones and menstrual cycle lengths with age." *Menopause.* 2005; 12: 567–577.

Fitzpatrick, L.A.; Pace, C.; et al. "Comparison of regimens containing oral micronized progesterone or medroxyprogesterone acetate on quality of life in postmenopausal women : a cross-sectional survey." *J of Women's Health and Gender-based Medicine.* 2000; 9(4): 381–387.

Formby, B.; Wiley, T.S. "Progesterone inhibits growth and induces apoptosis in breast cancer cells: Inverse effects on Bcl-2 and p53." *Ann Clin Lab Sci.* 1998; 28(6): 360–369.

Freeman, E.W.; Purdy, R.H.; Coutifaris, C.; Rickels, K.; Paul, S.M. "Anxiolytic metabolites of progesterone: correlation with mood and performance measures following oral progesterone administration to healthy female volunteers." *Neuroendocrinology.* 1993 Oct; 58(4): 478–84.

Gerhard, M., et al. "Estradiol therapy combined with progesterone; endothelium-dependent vasodilation in postmenopausal women." *Circulation.* 1998; 98(12): 1158–1163.

Gillet, J., et al. "Induction of amenorrhea during hormone replacement therapy: Optimal micronized progesterone dose. A multicenter study." *Maturitas.* 1994; 19: 103–115.

Gilson, G., et al. "A perspective on HRT for Women: Picking Up the Pieces After the Women's Health Initiative Trial, Part 2." *Intern Jour of Pharmaceutical Compounding.* 2003; 7(5): 330–338.

Gruber, D.M.; Sator, M.O.; et al. "Progesterone and neurology." *Gynecol Endocrin.* 1999; 13(Suppl4): 41–45.

Gulinello, M, et al. "Anxiogenic effects of neurosteroid exposure: sex differences and altered GABAA receptor pharmacology in adult rats." *Jour Pharmacol Exp Ther.* 2003; 305(2): 541–548.

Haffner, S., et al. "Endogenous sex hormones: impact on lipids, lipoproteins, and insulin." *Am J Med.* 1995; 98(1A): 40S-47S.

Hanaway, P. "Hormone essentials: Personalizing diagnosis and treatment." Module I, Anti-Aging and Regenerative Medicine Fellowship; Las Vegas, NV; Dec. 10–12, 2007.

Hargrove, J., et al. "Menopause." *Med Clin North Amer.* 1995; 79: 1337–1356.

Henderson, B., et al. "Estrogen replacement therapy and protection form acute MI." *Am J Obstet Gynecol.* 1988; 159: 312–317.

Hermsmeyer, R.K.; Rajesh, G.; Mishra, D.P.; et al. "Prevention of coronary hyperactivity in preatherogenic menopausal rhesus monkeys by transdermal progesterone." *Arterioscler Thromb Vasc Biol.* 2004; 24: 955–961.

Hermsmeyer, K.; Miyagawa, K.; et al. "Reactivity-based coronary vasospasm independent of atherosclerosis in rhesus monkeys." *J Am Coll Card.* 1997; 29(3): 671–80.

Herzog, A.G. "Intermittent progesterone therapy and frequency of complex partial seizures in women with menstrual disorders." *Neurology.* 1986 Dec; 36(12): 1607–10.

Jette, N.; Morrell, M.J. "Sex-steroid hormones in women with epilepsy." *The Female Patient.* 2004; 29(7): 23–29.

Kalkoff, R., et al. "Metabolic effects of progesterone." *J Obstect Gynecol.* 1982; 142–146, 735–738.

Khaw, K., et al. "Fasting plasma glucose levels and endogenous androgens in non-diabetic postmenopausal women." *Clin Sci.* 1991; 80(3): 199–203.

Kliman, H.B.; Keefe, C.L. "Route of progesterone affects rates of endometrial gland dyssynchrony in donor-egg patients undergoing mock cycles." http://info.med.yale.edu/obgyn/kliman/infertility/abstracts/Prog.html accessed 2/23/05.

Kojima, K., et al. "Progesterone inhibits apolipoprotein-mediated cellular lipid release: A putative mechanism for the decrease of high-density lipoprotein." *Biochim Biophy Acta.* 2001: 1532: 173–184.

Laux, M. *Natural Woman, Natural Menopause.* 1997; New York: HarperCollins, 20, 75–76.

Le Melledo, J., et al. "Role of progesterone and other neuroactive steroids in anxiety disorders." *Expert Rev Neuroter.* 2004; 4(5): 851–860.

Lee, J. *What Your Doctor May Not Tell You About Menopause.* 1996; New York: Warner, 88.

Leonetti, H.B.; Longo, S.; Anasti, J.N. "Topical progesterone cream for vasomotor symptoms and post-menopausal bone loss." *Obstet Gyneol.* 1999; 94: 225–228.

Levine, H., et al. "Comparison of the pharmacokinetics of crinone 8% administered vaginally versus Prometrium administered orally in postmenopausal women." *Fertil Steril.* 2000; 73: 516–521.

Luck, M., et al. "Ascorbic acid and fertility." *Biol Reproduc.* 1995; 52: 262–266.

Majewska, M., et al. "Steroid hormone metabolites are barbiturate-like modulators of the GABA receptor." *Science.* 1986; 232: 1004.

Manvais-Jarvis, P., et al. "Progesterone and progestins: a general overview." *Progesterone and Progestins.* 1983; New York: Rave Press, p. 1–16.

Martin, V.T.; Behbehani, M. "Ovarian hormones and migrane headache: understanding mechanisms and pathogenesis." *Headache.* 2006; 46(1): 2–23.

Martorano, J.T.; Ahlgrimm, M.; Colbert, T. "Differentiating between natural progesterone and synthetic progestins: clinical implications for premenstrual syndrome and perimenopause management." *Comrp Ther.* 1998 Jun-Jul; 24(6–7): 336–9.

Maurer, M.; Trajanoski, Z.; et al. "Differential gene expression profile of glucocorticoids, testosterone, and dehydroepiandrosterone in human cells." *Horm Metab Res.* 2001; 2(12):691–5.

McAuley, J., et al. "Oral administration of micronized progesterone; a review and more experience." *Pharmacotherapy.* 1996; 16(3): 453–457.

Melton, L., et al. "Progestins reverse some of the effects of estrogen." *TEM.* 2000; 11(2): 69–71.

Miles, R.A.; Paulson, R.J.; Lobo, R.A.; Press, M.A.; Dahmoush, L.; Sauer, M.B. "Pharmacokinetics and endometrial tissue levels of progesterone after administration by intramuscular and vaginal routes: a comparative study." *Fertility and Sterility.* 1995; 62: 485–490.

Minshall, R.D.; Miyagawa, K.; Chadwick, C.; et al. "In vitro modulation of primate coronary vascular muscle cell reactivity by ovarian steroid hormones." *The FASEB Journal.* 1998; 12: 1419–1429.

Minshall, R.; Pavcnik, D.; et al. "Nongenomic vasodilator action of progesterone on primate coronary arteries." *J Appl Physiol.* 2002; 92:701–708.

Minshall, R., et al. "Ovarian steroid protection against coronary artery hyperreactivity in rhesus monkeys." *J. Clin Endocrinol Metab.* 1998; 83(2): 649–659.

Minshall, R.D.; Pavcnik, D.; et al. "Progesterone regulation of vascular thromboxane A2 receptors in rhesus monkeys." *Am J Physiol Heart Circ Physiol.* 2001; 281: H1498–1507.

Miodrg, A., et al. "Sex hormones and the female urinary tract." *Drugs.* 1988; 36(4): 491–504.

Mircioiu, C.; Perju, A.; et al. "Pharmacokinetics of progesterone in postmenopausal women." *Eur J of Drug Metab and Pharmacokinetics.* 1998; 23: 397–401.

Miyagawa, K., et al. "Medroxyprogesterone interferes wit ovarian steroid proteciton against coronary vasospasm." *Nat Med.* 1997; 3: 324–327.

Molloy, E.J.; O'Neill, A.J.; et al. "Sex-specific alterations in neutrophil apoptosis: the role of estradiol and progesterone." *Blood.* 2003; 102(7): 2653–9.

Monjo, M.; Rodriguez, A.M.; et al. "Direct effects of testosterone, 17 beta-estradiol, and progesterone on adrenergic regulation in cultured brown adipocytes: potential mechanism for gender-dependent thermogenesis." *Endocrinology.* 2003; 144(11): 4923–30.

Montplaisir, J.; Lorrain, J.; et al. "Sleep in menopause : differential effects of two forms of hormone replacement therapy." *Menopause: The Journal of the North American Menopause Society.* 2001; 8(1): 10–16.

Ottosson, U., et al. "Oral progesterone and estrogen/progestogen therapy, effects of natural and synthetic hormones on subfractions of HDL cholesterol and liver proteins." *ACTA Obstet Gynecol Scand.* 1984; (Suppl): 127–137.

Ottoson, U., et al. "Subfractions of high-density lipo-protein cholesterol during estrogen replacement therapy: A comparison between progestogens and natural progesterone." *Journal of Obstetrics and Gynecology.* 1985; 151: 746–750.

Panth, M., et al. "Effect of vitamin A supplementation on plasma progesterone and estradiol levels during pregnancy." *Int J Vit Nutr Res.* 1991; p. 61.

Plu-Beureau, G.; Le, M.G.; et al. "Percutaneous progesterone use and risk of breast cancer : results from a French cohort study of premenopausal women with benign breast disease." *Cancer Detection and Prevention.* 1999; 23(4): 290–296.

Prior, J., et al. "Progesterone as a bone-tropic hormone." *Endocrine Reviews.* 1990; 11: 386–398.

Project AWARE. "Synthetic Progestins and Natural Progesterone, A Pharmacist Explores the differences." http://www.project-aware.org/Resource/articlearchives/differences.shtml

Ren, K.; Wei, F.; et al. "Progesterone attenuates persistent inflammatory hyperalgesia in female rats: involvement of spinal NMDA receptor mechanisms." *Brain Research.* 2000; 865: 272–277.

Rodriguez, I.; Kilborn, M.J.; Liu, X.X.; et al. "Drug-induced QT prolongation in women during the menstrual cycle." *JAMA.* 2001; 285: 1322–1326.

Rosano, G., et al. "Natural progesterone, but not medroxyprogesterone acetate, enhances the beneficial effect of estrogen on exercise-induced myocardial ischemia in postmenopausal women." *Jour Amer Coll Cardiol.* 2000; 36: 2154–2159.

Ross, R., et al. "Effect of hormone replacement therapy on breast cancer risk: estrogen versus estrogen plus progestin." *J Natl Cancer Inst.* 1992; (4): 328–332.

Rouzier, N. "Thyroid replacement therapy." *Longevity and Preventive Medicine Symposium.* 2002; 2, 12–14.

Schairer, C., et al. "Menopausal estrogen and estrogen-progestin replacement therapy and breast cancer risk." *JAMA.* 2000; 283: 485–491.

Schedlowski, M., et al. "Acute psychological stress increases plasma levels of cortisol, prolactin and thyroid stimulating hormone." *Life Sciences.* 1992; 50: 1201–1205.

Schmidt, M.; Renner, C.; Loffler, G. "Progesterone inhibits glucocorticoid-dependent aromatase induction in human adipose fibroblasts." *J Endocrinol.* 1998; 158(3): 401–407.

Simoncini, T., et al. "Differential signal transduction of progesterone and medroxyprogesterone acetate in human endothelial cells." *Endocrinology.* 2004; 145(12): 5745–5756.

Sinatra, S. *Heart Sense for Women.* 2000; Washington D.C.: LifeLine Press, 108, 219.

Stanczyk, F.Z.; et al. "Percutaneous administration of progesterone: blood levels and endometrial protaction." *Menopause.* 2005; 12(2): 232–237.

Stefanick, M., et al. "Estrogen, progestogens and cardiovascular risk: review of PEPPI trial." *J Repro Med.* 1999; 44(2suppl): 221–226.

Stein, D. "The case for progesterone." *Ann NY Acad Sci.* 2005; 1052: 152–159.

Stephenson, K.; Price C.; Neuenschwander, P.; Kurdowska, A.; et al. "Topical progesterone cream does not increase thrombotic and inflammatory factors in postmenopausal women." *Blood.* 2004; 104(11): 414b-415b.

Sternberg, W.F.; Chesler, E.J.; et al. "Acute progesterone can recruit sex-specific neurochemical mechanisms mediating swim stress-induced and kappa-opioid analgesia in mice." *Horm Behav.* 2004; 46(4): 467–473.

Sumino, H., et al. "Hormone replacement therapy decreases insulin resistance and lipid metabolism in Japanese postmenopausal women with impaired and normal glucose tolerance." *Horm Res.* 2003; 60(3): 134–142.

Taylor, D. "Perimenstrual symptoms and syndromes: Guidelines for symptom management and self care." *Obstetrics and Gynecology.* 2005; 5(5): 228–241.

Trainor, B.C.; Bird, I.M.; et al. "Variation in aromatase activity in the medial preoptic area and plasma progesterone is associated with the onset of paternal behavior." *Neuroendocrinology.* 2003; 78(1): 36–44.

Unger, J.; Cady, R.; Farmer-Cady, K. "Migrane headaches, part 3: Hormonal factors." *The Female Patient.* 2003; 28(7): 31–34.

Vliet, E. "An approach to preimenopausal migraine." *Menopause Management.* 1995; Nov/Dec: 25–33.

Vliet, E., et al. "New insights on hormones and mood." *Menopause Management.* 1993; June/July: 140–146, 227.

Vliet, E. *Women Weight and Hormones.* 2001; New York: M. Evans & Company, 25, 93, 95–96, 99–100.

Waddell, B.J.; O'Leary, P.C. "Distribution and metabolism of topically applied progesterone in a rat model." *Journal of Steroid Biochemistry & Molecular Biology.* 2002; 80: 449–455.

Wakatsuki, A., et al. "Effect of medroxyprogesterone acetate on endothelium-dependent vasodilation in postmenopausal women receiving estrogen." *Circulation.* 2001; 104: 1773–1778.

Wilson, M.E. "Premature elevation in serum insulin-like growth factor-I advances first ovulation in rhesus monkeys." *Journal of Endocrinology.* 1998; 158: 247–257.

The Writing Group for the Postmenopausal Estrogen/Progestin Interventions (PEPI) Trial. "Effects of estrogen or estrogen/progestin regimens on heart disease risk factors in postmenopausal women." *JAMA.* 1995; 273: 199–208.

Xilouri, M.; Papazafiri, P. "Anti-apoptotic effects of allopregnanolone on P19 neurons." *Eur J Neurosci.* 2006; 23(1): 43–54.

## ESTROGEN/PROGESTERONE RATIO

Bland, J. "Introduction to neuroendocrine disorders." *Functional Medicine Approaches to Endocrine Disturbances of Aging.* 2001; Gig Harbor, Washington: The Functional Medicine Institute, 57, 71.

Collins, J. *What's Your Menopause Type.* 2000; Roseville, CA: Prima Health, 79.

Vliet, E. *Women Weight and Hormones.* 2001; New York: M. Evans & Company, 25, 97–98, 129.

## TESTOSTERONE

Almeida, O.P. "Sex playing with the mind. Effects of oestrogen and testosterone on mood and cognition. *Arch Neuropsysch.* 1999; 57(3A): 701–706.

Apperloo, M.J.; Van Der Stege, J.G.; Hoek, A.; et al. "In the mood for sex: The value of androgens." *J Sex Marital Ther.* 2003; 29(2): 87–102.

Bachmann, G.; Bancroft, J.; Braustein, G.; et al. "Female androgen insufficiency: The Princeton consensus statement on definition, classification, and assessment." *Fertil Steril.* 2002; 77(4): 660–665.

Bland, J. "Introduction to neuroendocrine disorders." *Functional Medicine Approaches to Endocrine Disturbances of Aging.* 2001; Gig Harbor, Washington: The Functional Medicine Institute, 57, 71, 74.

Brincat, M., et al. "Sex hormones and skin collagen content in postmenopausal woman." *Br Med J.* 1983; 287(6402): 1337–1338.

Burger, H.G.; Dudley, E.C.; Dennerstein, L.; Hopper, J.L. "A prospective longitudinal study of serum testosterone, dehydroepiandrosterone sulfate, and sex hormone-binding globulin levels through the menopause transition." *J Clin Endocrinol Metab.* 2000; 85(8): 2832–2838.

Davis, S.R.; Tran, J. "Testosterone influences libido and well being in women." *Trends Endocrinol Metab.* 2001; 2(1): 33–37.

Davis, S., et al. "Use of androgens in postmenopausal women." *Curr Opin Obstet Gynecol.* 1997; 9(3): 177–180.

Donato, G.B.; Fuchs, S.C.; Oppermann, K. "Association between menopause status and central adiposity measured at different cutoffs of waist circumference and waist-to-hip ratio." *Menopause.* 2006; 13(2): 280–285.

Ehrenreish, H.; Halaris, A.; Ruether, E.; et al. "Psychoendocrine sequelae of chronic testosterone deficiency." *J Psychiatr Res.* 1999; 33(5): 379–387.

English, K.M.; Steeds, R.P.; Jones, T.H.; et al. "Low-dose transdermal testosterone therapy improves agina threshold in men with chronic stable angina." *Circulation.* 2000; 120: 1906–1911.

Fink, G.; Sumner, B.E.; McQueen, J.K.; et al. "Sex steroid control of mood, mental state and memory." *Clin Exp Pharmacol Physiol.* 1998; 25(10): 764–775.

Hanaway, P. "Hormone essentials: Personalizing diagnosis and treatment." Module I, Anti-Aging and Regenerative Medicine Fellowship; Las Vegas, NV; Dec. 10–12, 2007.

Janssen, I.; Powell, L.H.; et al. "Development of the metabolic syndrome through menopause: The Study of Women's Health Across the Nation (SWAN)." *Circulation.* 2007; 115(8).

Jensen, M.D. "Andorgen effect on body composition and fat metabolism." *Mayo Clin Proc.* 2000; 75(Suppl): S65–S68.

Laux, M. *Natural Woman, Natural Menopause.* 1997; New York: HarperCollins; 20, 119.

Maurer, M.; Trajanoski, Z.; Frey, G.; et al. "Differential gene expression profile of glucocorticoids, testosterone, and dehydroepiandrosterone in human cells." *Horm Metab Res.* 2001; 33(12): 691–695.

Moller, J.; Einfeldt H. *Testosterone Treatment of Cardiovascular Diseases.* 1984; Berlin, Germany: Springer Verlag.

Monjo, M.; Rodriguez, A.M.; et al. "Direct effects of testosterone, 17 beta-estradiol, and progesterone on adrenergic regulation in cultured brown adipocytes: potential mechanism for gender-dependent thermogenesis." *Endocrinology.* 2003; 144(11): 4923–30.

Notelovitz, M. "Hot flashes and androgens: A biological rationale for clinical practice." *Mayo Clin Proc.* 2004; 79(4 Suppl): S8–S13. *Nutrition and Healing Newsletter.* 1995; Vol 11, No. 12.

Persky, H., et al. "Plasma testosterone level and sexual behavior of couples." *Arch Sex Behav.* 1978; 7(3): 157–173.

Rohr, U.D. "The impact of testosterone imbalance on depression and women's health." *Maturitas.* 2002; 41(Suppl): S25–S46.

Sand, R., et al. "Exogenous androgens in postmenopausal women." *Am J of Med.* 1995; 98 (1A).

Sari, M.; Van Anders, M.A.; Hampson, E. "Waist-to-hip ratio is positively associated with bioavailable testosterone but negatively associated with sexual desire in healthy premenopausal women." *Psychosomatic Medicine.* 2005; 67: 246–250.

Sarrel, P., et al. "Cardiovascular aspects of androgens in women." *Semin Reprod Endocrinol.* 1998; 16(2): 121–128.

Sarrel, P., et al. "Vasodilator effects of estrogen are not diminished by androgen in postmenopausal women." *Fertil Steril.* 1997; 68(6): 1125–1127.

Schmidt, J., et al. "Other anti-androgens." *Dermatology.* 1998; 196(1): 153–157.

Shippen, E. *Testosterone Syndrome.* 1998; New York: M. Evans & Company Inc., 145, 152.

Sowers, M.F.; Beebe, J.L.; McConnell, D.; et al. "Testosterone concentrations in women aged 25–50 years: Associations with lifestyle, body composition, and ovarian status." *Am J Epidemiol.* 2001; 153: 256–264.

Springer-Verlag, S. *Testosterone: Action, Deficiency, Substitution.* 1998: Berlin, 299.

Surrel, P., et al. "Cardiovascular aspects of androgens in women." *Semin Repro Endocrinol.* 1998; 16(2):121–128.

Vliet, E. *Women Weight and Hormones.* 2001; New York: M. Evans & Company, 25, 108–110.

Wabitsch, M.; Hauner, H.; Heinze, E.; Bockmann, A.; Benz, R. "Body fat distribution and steroid hormone concentrations in obese adolescent girls before and after weight reduction." *J Clin Endocrinol Metab.* 1995 Dec; 80(12): 3469–75.

Weber, B.; Lewicka, S.; Deuschle, M.; et al. "Testosterone, androstenidione and dihydrotestosterone concentrations and elevated in female patients with major depression." *Psychoneuroendocrinology.* 2000; 25(8): 765–771.

Worboys, S.; Kotsopoulos, D.; Teede, H.; McGrath, B.; Davis, S.R. "Evidence that parenteral testosterone therapy may improve endothelium-dependent and -independent vasodilation in postmenopausal women already receiving estrogen." *J Clin Endocrinol Metab.* 2001; 86(1): 158–161.

## DHEA

Ahlgrimm, M. *The HRT Solution.* 1999; New York: Avery Publishing, 22, 28.

Arlt, W.; Callies, F.; Can Clijmen, J.C.; Koehler, I.; Reincke, M.; Bidlingmaier, M.; et al. "Dehydroepiandrosterone replacement in women with adrenal insufficiency." *New England Journal of Medicine.* 1999; 341(14): 1013–1020.

Barbieri, R., et al. "Cotinine and nicotine inhibit human fetal adrenal 11, beta-hydroxylase." *J Clin Endocrinol Metab.* 1989; 69: 1221–1224.

Barrett-Conner, E., et al. "A prospective study of dehydroepiandrosterone sulfate, mortality and cardiovascular disease." *NEJM.* 1986; 37(9): 1035.

Brownstein, D. *Overcoming Thyroid Disorders.* 2002; West Bloomfield, MI: Medical Alternatives Press, 8, 140.

Buffington, C., et al. "Case report: amelioration of insulin resistance in diabetes with dehydroepiandrosterone." *Amer Jour Med Sci.* 1993; 306(5): 320–324.

Casson, P.R.; Andersen, R.N.; Herrod, H.G.; et al. "Oral dehydroepiandrosterone in physiologic doses modulates immune function in postmenopausal women." *Am J Obstet Gynecol.* 1993; 169(6): 1536–1539.

Casson, P.R.; Faquin, L.C.; Stentz, F.B. "Replacement of dehydroepiandrosterone enhances T-lynphocyte insulin binding in postmenopausal women." *Fertility and Sterility.* 1995; 63(5): 1027–1031.

De Bruin, V.M.; Vieira, M.C.; Rocha, M.N.; Viana, G.S. "Cortisol and dehydroepiandrosterone sulfate plasma levels and their relationship to aging, cognitive function, and dementia." *Brain Cogn.* 2002; 50(2): 316–323.

Gordon, G., et al. "Reduction of atherosclerosis by administration of dehydroepiandrosterone. A study of the hypercholesterolemic New Zealand white rabbit with aortic internal injury." *J. Clin Invest.* 1988; 82: 712.

Khorram, O., et al. "Activation of immune function by dehydroepiandrosterone (DHEA) in age-advanced men." *Jour Gerontol A Biol Sci Med Sci.* 1997; 52(1): 1–7.

Labrie, F.; Diamond, P.; Cusan, L.; Gomez, J.L.; Belander, A.; Candas, B. "Effect of 12-month dehydroepuandrosterone replacement therapy on bone, vagina, and endometrium in postmenopausal women." *J Clin Endocrinol Metab.* 1997; 82(10): 3498–3505.

Legrain, S.; Massien, C.; Lahlou, N.; et al. "Dehydroepiandrosterone replacement administration: pharmacokinetic and pharmacodynamic studies in healthy elderly subjects." *Clin Endocrinol Metab.* 2000; 85(9): 3208–3217.

Lieberman, S. *The Real Vitamin and Mineral Book.* New York: Avery Publishing, 1997; 216, 220.

Morales, A.J.; Nolan, J.J.; Nelson, J.C.; Yen, S.S. "Effects of replacement dose of dehydroepiandrosterone in men and women of advancing age." *J Clin Endocrinol Metab.* 1994; 78(6): 1360–1367. Erratum in: *J Clin Endocrinol Metab.* 1995; 80(9): 2799.

Nawata, H., et al. "Aromatase in bone cell: association with osteoporosis in postmenopausal women." *Jour Steroid Biochem Mol Biol.* 1995; 53(1–6): 1650–1674.

Schmidt, P.J.; Daly, R.C.; Bloch, M.; et al. "Dehydroepiandrosterone monotherapy in midlife-onset major and minor depression." *Arch Gen Psychiatry.* 2005; 62: 154–162.

Stomati, M.; Monteleone. P.; Casaros. E.; Quirici, B.; Puccetti, S.; Bernardi, F.; Genazzani, A.D.; Rovati, L.; Luisi, M.; Genazzani, A.R. "Six month oral dehydroespiandrosterone supplementation in early and late postmenopause." *Dynecol Endocrinol.* 2000; 14: 342–363.

Villareal, D.T.; Holloszy, J.O. "Effect of DHEA on abdominal fat and insulin action in elderly women and men." *JAMA.* 2004; 292: 2243–2248.

Watson, R., et al. "Dehydroepiandrosterone and diseases of aging." *Drugs Aging.* 1996; 9(4): 274–291.

Yamaguchi, Y., et al. "Reduced serum dehydroepiandrosterone levels in diabetic patients with hyperinsulinaemia." *Endocrinol (Oxf).* 1998; 49(3): 377–383.

Yeh, J., et al. "Nicotine and cotinine inhibit rat testes androgen biosynthesis in vitro." *J Steroid Biochem.* 1989; 33(4A): 627–630.

Yen, S., et al. "Increased risk of endometrial carcinoma among users of conjugated estrogens." *NEJM*.1975; 293(23): 1170–1176.

Yen, S.S.; Morales, A.J.; Khorram, O. "Replacement of DHEA in aging men and women. Potential remedial effects." *Ann NY Acad Sci*. 1995; 774: 128–142.

Young, D. "Pregnenolone." 2000; Salem, UT: Essential Science Publishing.

## CORTISOL

Allison, T., et al. "Medical and economic costs of psychologic distress in patients with coronary artery disease." *Mayo Clin Proc*. 1995; 70(8): 734–742.

Antoni, M., et al. "Elevated basal cortisol levels and attenuated ACTH and cortisol responses to a behavioral challenge in women with metastatic breast cancer." *Psychoneuroendocrinology*. 1996; 21(4): 361–374.

Armanini, D., et al. *Steroids*. 2004; 69(11–12): 763–766.

Barker, J., et al. "The naturopathic approach to adrenal dysfunction." *Townsend Letter*. 2005; Feb/March: 59–62.

Baum, A.; Cohen, L.; Hall, M. "Control and intrusive memories as possible determinants of chronic stress." *Psychosom Med*. 1993; 55(3): 274–286.

Beer, J.; Beer, J. "Burnout and stress, depression and self-esteem of teachers." *Psychol Rep*. 1992; 71(3 Pt 2): 1331–1336.

Black, P.H. "The inflammatory reponse is an integral part of the stress response: Implications for atherosclerosis, insulin resistance, type II diabetes and metabolic syndrome X." *Brain Behav Immun*. 2003; 17(5): 350–364.

Black, P.H.; Garbutt, L.D. "Stress, inflammation and cardiovascular disease." *J Psychosom Res*. 2002; 52(1): 1–23.

Bland, J. "Introduction to neuroendocrine disorders." *Functional Medicine Approaches to Endocrine Disturbances of Aging*. 2001; Gig Harbor, Washington: The Functional Medicine Institute, 57, 121.

Bliel, M.E.; McCaffery, J.M.; et al. "Anger-related personality traits and carotid artery atherosclerosis in untreated hypertensive men."

Brody, S., et al. "A randomized controlled trial of high dose ascorbic acid for reduction of blood pressure, cortisol, and subjective responses to psychological stress." *Psychopharmacology (Berl)*. 2002; 159(3): 319–324.

Buljevac, D., et al. "Self reported stressful life events and exacerbations in multiple sclerosis: prospective study." *BJM*. 2003; 327(7416): 646.

Camacho, A.; Dimsdale, J.E. "Platelets and psychiatry: lessons learned from old and new studies."

Carlson, L., et al. "Relationships among cortisol (CRT), dehydroepiandrosterone-sulfate (DHEAS), and memory in a longitudinal study of healthy elderly men and women." *Neurobiol Aging*. 1999; 20(3): 315–324.

Chrousos, G.P.; Gold, P.A. "A healthy body in healthy mind—and vice versa—the damaging power of 'uncontrollable' stress." *The Journal of Clinical Endocrinology & Metabolism*. 1998; 83(6): 1842–1845.

Cohen, S. "Psychological stress and susceptibility to upper respiratory infections." *Amer Jour Respire Crit Care Med*. 1995; 152(4 Pt.2): 53–58.

Dantzer, R. "Cytokine-induced sickness behavior: A neuroimmune response to activation of innate immunity." *Eur J Pharmacol*. 2004; 500: 399–411.

Dedert, E.A.; Studta, J.L.; Weissbecher, I.; et al. "Religiosity may help preserve the cortisol rhythm in women with stress-related illness." *Int J Psych in Med*. 2004; 34(1): 61–77.

Delarue, J., et al. "Fish oil prevents the adrenal activation elicited by mental stress in healthy men." *Diabetes Metab*. 2003; 29(3): 289–295.

Elenkov, I.J.; Webster, E.L.; Torpy, D.J.; et al. "Stress, corticotropin-releasing hormone, glucocorticoids, and the immune/inflammatory response: acute and chronis effects." *Annals of NY Acad of Sciences*. 1999; 876: 1–13.

Elenkov, I.J.; Chrousos, G.P. "Stress, cytokine patterns and susceptibility to disease." *Bailliere's Clinical Endocri and Metabl*. 1999; 13: 583–595.

Elenkov, I.J. "Systemic stress-induced Th2 shift and its clinical implications." *Interna Revi of Neurobiology*. 2002; 52: 163–186.

Epel, E.; Blackburn, E.; Lin, J.; et al. "Accelerated telomere shortening in response to life stress." *PNASA*. 2004; 101: 17312–17315.

Eskandari, F.; Mistry, S.; Martinez, P.E.; et al. "Younger, Premenopausal women with major depressive disorder have more abdominal fat and increased serum levels of prothrombotic factors: Implications for greater cardiovascular risk. The POWER Study." *Metabolism Clinical and Experimental*. 2005; 54: 918–924.

Everly, G.S. "The development of a stress scale to assess behavioral health factors." The Everly Stress and Symptom Inventory. *Advances in Health Education*. 1989; 2: 71–86.

Ferrari, E., et al. "Age-related changes of the adrenal secretory pattern: possible role in pathological brain aging." *Brain Res Brain Res Rev*. 2001; 37(1–3): 294–300.

Goldman M.D. *Brain Fitness*. 1999; New York: Random House.

Gozansky, W.S.; Lynn, J.S.; Laudenslager, M.L.; et al. "Salivary cortisol determined by enzyme immunoassay is preferable to serum total cortisol for assessment of dynamic hypothalamic-pituitary-adrenal axis activity." *Clinical Endocrinology*. 2005; 63: 336–341.

Griffin, M.G.; Resick, P.A.; Yehuda, R. "Enhanced cortisol suppression following dexamethasone administration in domestic violence survivors." *American Journal of Psychiatry*. 2005; 162: 1192–1199.

Hawkley, L.C.; Burleson, M.H.; et al. "Cardiovascular and endocrine reactivity in older females: intertask consistency." *Psychophysiology*. 2001; 38: 863–872.

Heim, C.; Ehlert, U.; Hanker, J.P.; Hellhammer, D.H. "Abuse-related posttraumatic stress disorder and alterations of the hypothalamic-pituitary-adrenal axis in women with chronic pelvic pain." *Psychosom Med*. 1998; 60: 309–318.

Heim, C.; Newport, D.J.; et al. "The role of early adverse experience and adulthood stress in the prediction of neuroendocrine stress reactivity in women: a multiple regression analysis." *Depression and Anxiety*. 2002; 15: 117–125.

Heller, L. *The Essentials of Herbal Care Part II*. 2000; San Clemente, CA: Metagenics, Inc., 1144–1145.

Janice, K.; Kiecolt-Glaser, PhD; Timothy, J.; Loving, PhD; Jeffrey, R.; Stowell, PhD; Williams, B.; Malarkey, MD; Stanley, Lemeshow, PhD; Stephanie, L.; Dickinson, MAS; Ronald, Glaser, PhD. "Hostile marital interactions, proinflammatory cytokine production, and would healing." *Arch Gen Psychiatry*. 2005; 62: 1377–1384.

Jezova, D., et al. "Reduction of rise in blood pressure and cortisol release during stress by Ginkgo biloba extract (EGb 761) in healthy volunteers." *Jour Physiol Pharmacol*. 2002; 53(3): 337–348.

Karten, Y.J.G.; Olariu, A.; Cameron, H.A. "Stress in early life inhibits neurogenesis in adulthood." *Trends in Neuroscience*. 2005; 28(4): 171.

Kelly, G. "Nutritional and botanical interventions to assist with the adaptation to stress." *Alern Med Rev*. 1999; 4(4); 249–265.

Kelly, G. "Rhodiola rosea: a possible plant adaptogen." *Alern Med Rev*. 2001; 6(3): 293–302.

Kiecolt-Glaser, J.K.; Loving, T.J.; Stowell, J.R.; Malarkey, W.B.; et al. "Hostile marital interactions, proinflammatory cytokine production and wound healing." *Archives of General Psychiatry*. 2005; 62(12): 1377–1384.

Krahenbuhl, S., et al. "Kinetics and dynamics of orally administered 18 beta-glycyrrhetinic acid in humans." *Jour Clin Endocrin Metab*. 1994; 78: 581–585.

Krause, N.; Shaw, B.A.; Cairney, J. "A descriptive epidemiology of lifetime trauma and the physical health status of older adults." *Psychol Aging*. 2004; 19(4): 637–648.

Krause, N. "Exploring age differences in the stress-buffering function of social support." *Psychol Aging*. 2005; 20(4): 714–717.

Kudielka, B.M.; Schmidt-Reinwald, A.K.; Hellhammer, D.H.; Kirschbaum, C. "Psychological and endocrine responses to psychological stress and dexamethasone/corticotrophin-releasing hormone in healthy postmenopausal women and young controls: the impact of age and a two-week estradiol treatment." *Neuroendocrinol*. 1999; 70: 422–430.

Kunz-Ebrecht, S.R.; Mohamed-Ali, V.; Fledman, P.J.; et al. "Cortisol responses to mild psychological stress are inversely associated with proinflammatory cytokines." *Brain Behav Immun*. 2003; 17(5): 373–383.

LaValle, J. "Current concepts in metabolic regulation: the role of nutrients and novel agents." *Module IV, Anti-Aging and Functional Medicine Fellowship.* 2007; Sept 14–16: Detroit, MI.

Lea, R., et al. "Psychological influences on the irritable bowel syndrome." *Minerva Med.* 2004; 95(5): 443–450.

Lee, A., et al. "Stress and depression: possible links to neuron death in the hippocampus." *Bipolar Disord.* 2002; 4(2): 117–128.

Lerner, J.S.; Gonzalez, R.M.; Dahl, R.E.; et al. "Facial expressions of emotion reveal neuroendocrine and cardiovascular stress responses." *Biol Psychiatr.* 2005; 58: 743–750.

Leucken, L.J.; Suarez, E.C.; et al. "Stress in employed women: impact of marital status and children at home on neurohormone output and home strain." *Psychosom Med.* 1997; 59: 352–359.

Locke, G., et al. "Psychosocial factors are linked to functional gastrointestinal disorders: a population based nested case-control study." *Amer Jour Gastroenterol.* 2004; 99(2): 350–357.

Lovallo, W.R.; Gerin, W. "Psychophysiological reactivity: mechanisms and pathways to cardiovascular disease."

Luecken, L.J.; Rodiriguez, A.P.; Appelhans, B.M. "Cardiovascular stress responses in young adulthood associated with family-of-origin relationship experiences." *Psychosomatic Medicine.* 2005; 67: 513–521.

Lupien, S.J.; De Leon, M.; De Santi, S.; Convit, A.; Tarshish, C.; Nair, N.P.V.; Thakur, M.; McEwen, B.S.; Hauger, R.L.; Meaney, M.J. "Cortisol levels during human aging predict hippocampal atrophy and memory deficits." *Nature Neuroscience.* 1998; 1(12): 69–73.

MacLean, C., et al. "Effects of the Transcendental Meditation program on adaptive mechanisms: changes in hormone levels and responses to stress after 4 months of practice." *Psychoneuroendocrinology.* 1997; 22(4): 277–295.

Medical Letter on the CDC & FDA (2005, June 5). *Alzheimer disease; up-regulation of glutathione protects neurons against A-beta toxicity.* Alanta: 13.

Monteleone, P., et al. "Blunting by chronic phosphatidylserine administration of the stress-induced activation of the hypothalamo-pituitary-adrenal axis in healthy men." *Eur Jour Clin Pharmacol.* 1992; 42(4): 385–388.

Newcomer, J.; Selke, G.; Melson, A.; Hershey, T.; Craft, S.; Richards, K.; Alderson, A. "Decreased memory performance in healthy humans induced by stress-level cortisol treatment." *Archives of General Psychiatry.* 1999; 56: 527–533.

Nocerino, E., et al. "The aphrodisiac and adaptogenic properties of ginseng." *Fitoter Apia.* 2000; Aug 71 Suppl 1: 1–5.

Ohlin, B., et al. "Chronic psychosocial stress predicts long-term cardiovascular morbidity and mortality in middle-aged men." *Eur Heart Jour.* 2004; 25(10): 867–873.

Olson, M.B.; Krantz, D.S.; Kelsey, S.F.; et al. "Hostility scores are associated with increased risk of cardiovascular events in women undergoing coronary angiography: A report from the NHLBI-Sponsored Women's Ischemic Syndrome Evaluation (WISE) Study." *Psychosomatic Medicine.* 2005; 67: 546–552.

Padgett, D.A.; Glaser, R. "How stress influences the immune response." *Trends in Immunol.* 2003; 24: 444–448.

Papanicolaou, D.A.; Wilder, R.L.; et al. "The pathophysiologic roles of Interleukin-6 in human disease." *Ann Intern Med.* 1998; 128: 127–137.

Peters, E., et al. "Vitamin C supplementation attenuates the increase in circulating cortisol, adrenaline and anti-inflammatory polypeptides following ultramarathon running." *Int Jour Sports Med.* 2001; 22(7): 537–543.

Pruessner, J.C.; Hellhammer, D.H.; Kirschbaum, C. "Burnout, perceived stress and cortisol response to awakening." *Psychosom Med.* 1999; 61: 197–204.

Raber, J. "Detrimental effects of chronic hypothalamic-pituitary-adrenal axis activation. From obesity to memory deficits." *Mol Neurobiol.* 1998; 18(1): 1–22.

Reiche, E., et al. "Stress, depression, the immune system, and cancer." *Lancet Oncol.* 2004; 5(10): 617–625.

Rosick, E. "Cortisol, stress, and health." *Life Extension*. 2005; Dec.: 40–48.

Sapolsky, M. "Social status and health in humans and other animals." *Annual Review of Anthropology*. 2004; 33: 393–419.

Scott, L.; Salahuddin, F.; Cooney, J.; et al. "Differences in adrenal steroid profile in chronic fatigue syndrome, in depression, and in health." *J Affect Disord*. 1999; 54: 129–137.

Selye, H. *The Stress of Life*. Revised ed. 976; New York, NY: McGraw Hill.

Sephton, S.; Spiegel, D. "Circadian disruption in cancer: A neuroendocrine-immune pathway from stress to disease?" *Brain Behav Immun*. 2003; 17(5): 321–328.

Segerstrom, S.C.; Miller, G.E. "Psychological stress and the human immune system: A meta-analytic study of 30 years of inquiry." *Psych Bull*. 2004; 130(4): 601–630.

Sherline, Y.; Sanghavi, M.; Mintun, M.; Gado, M. "Depression duration but nor age predicts hippocampal volume loss in medical healthy women with recurrent major depression." *Journal of Neuroscience*. 1999; 19: 5034–5041.

Sherline, Y.; Gado, M.; Kraemer, H. "Untreated depression and hippocampal volume loss." *American Journal of Psychiatry*. 2003; 160: 1516.

Stones, A.; Groome, D.; Perry, D.; Hucklebridge, F.; Evans, P. "The effect of stress on salivary cortisol in panic disorder patients." *J Affect Disorders*. 1999; 52: 197–201.

Van der Kolk, B. "The psychobiology of post-traumatic stress disorder." *Journal of Clinical Psychiatr*. 1997; 58(9): 16–24.

Vedhara, K.; Hyde, J.; Gilchrist, I.D.; Tytherleigh, M.; Plummer, S. "Acute stress, memory, attention, and cortisol." *Psychoneuroendocrin*. 2000; 25: 535–549.

Vliet, E. *Women Weight and Hormones*. 2001; New York: M. Evans & Company, 25, 129, 140.

Vrijkotte, T.G.; Van Doornen, L.J.P.; et al. "Overcommitment to work is associated with changes in cardic sympathetic regulation."

Vrijkotte, T.G.; Van Doornen, S.J.P. "Work stress and metabolic and hemostatic risk factors."

Wilson, J. "Adrenal Fatigue," *Anti-Aging and Functional Medicine Fellowship: Module I*. 2007; December 10–12: Las Vegas, NV.

Wilson, J. *Adrenal Fatigue*. 2001; Petaluma, CA: Smart Publications.

Wilson, R., et al. "Proneness to psychological distress is associated with risk of Alzheimer's disease." *Neurology*. 2003; 61(11): 1479–1485.

Winter, H.; Irle, E. "Hippocampal volume in adult burn patients with and without post-traumatic stress disorder." *The American Journal of Psychiatry*. 2004; 161(12): 2194–2200.

Yehuda, R.; Golier, J.A.; Kaufman, S. "Circadian rhythm of salivary cortisol in holocaust survivors with and without PTSD." *American Journal of Psychiatr*. 2005; 162: 998–1000.

## PREGNENOLONE

Akwa, Y., et al. "Neurosteroids: biosynthesis, metabolism, and function of pregnenolone and dehydroepiandrosterone in the brain." *Jour Steroid Biochem Mol Biol*. 1991; 40(1–3): 71–81.

Alayo, W., et al. "Individual differences in cognitive aging: implication of pregnenolone sulfate." *Prog Neurobio*. 2002; 71(1): 43–48.

Darnaudery, M., et al. "The neurosteroid pregnenolone sulfate infused into the medical septum nucleus increased hippocampal aceteylcholine and spatial memory in rats." *Brain Res*. 2002; 951(2): 237–242.

DePeretti, E., et al. "Pattern of plasma pregnenolone sulfate levels in human from birth to adulthood." *Jour Clin Endocrinol Metab*. 1983; 57(3): 550–556.

George, M., et al. "CSF neuroactive steroids in affective disorders: pregnenolone, progesterone, and DBI." *Biol Psychiatry*. 1994; 35(10): 775–780.

Guth, L., et al. "Key role for pregnenolone in combination therapy that promotes recovery after spinal cord injury." *Proc Natl Acad Sci USA*. 1994; 91(25): 12308–12312.

Havlikova, H., et al. "Sex and age-related changes in epitestosterone in relation to pregnenolone sulfate and testosterone in normal subjects" *Jour Clin Endocrinology Met*. 2002; 87(5): 2225–2237.

Kaplan, J., et al. "Assessing the observed relationship between low cholesterol and violence-related mortality. Implications for suicide risk." *Ann NY Acad Sci*. 1997; 836: 57–80.

Labrie, F., et al. "Marked decline in serum concentrations of adrenal C19 sex steroid precursors and conjugated androgen metabolites during aging." *Jour Clin Endocrinol Metab.* 1997; 82(8): 2396–2402.

Mayo, W., et al. "Pregnenolone sulfate and aging of cognitive functions: behavioral, neurochemical, and morphological investigations." *Horm Behav.* 2001; 40(2): 215–217.

McGavack, T., et al. "The use of delta 5-pregnenolone in various clinical disorders." *Jour Clin Endocrinol Metabol.* 1951; 11(6): 559–577.

Ravaglia, G., et al. "Determinants of functional status in healthy Italian nonagenarians and centenarians: a comprehensive functional assessment by the instruments of geriatric practice." *Jour Amer Geriatr Soc.* 1997; 45(10): 1196–1202.

Roberts, E., et al. "Pregnenolone from Selye to Alzheimer's and a model of the pregnenolone sulfate binding site on the GABA receptor." *Biochemical Pharmacology.* 1995; (49)1: 1–16.

Steiger, A., et al. "Neurosteroid pregnenolone induces sleep-EEG changes in man compatible with inverse agonistic GABA receptor modulation." *Brain Res.* 1993; 615(2): 267–274.

Vallee, M., et al. "Role of pregnenolone, dehydroepiandrosterone and their sulfate esters on learning and memory in cognitive aging." *Brain Res Rev.* 2001; 37(1–2): 301–312.

Wu, F., et al. "Pregnenolone sulfate: a positive allosteric modulator at the N-methyl-D-aspartate receptor." *Mol Pharmacol.* 1991; 40(3): 333–336.

Yanick, P. *Prohormone Nutritio.* 1998; Montclair, NJ: Longevity Institute International, 358.

Young, D. *Pregnenolone.* 2000; Salem, UT: Essential Science Publishing.

## INSULIN

Bland, J. "Carbohydrate intolerance, insulin, DHEA and oxidative stress." *Nutritional Improvement of Health Outcomes The Inflammatory Disorders.* 1997; Gig Harbor, WA: The Institute For Functional Medicine, Inc., 81.

Bruning, P., et al. "Insulin resistance and breast cancer risk." *Int Jour Cancer.* 1992; 52(4): 511–516.

Cauley, J., et al. "Elevated serum estradiol and testosterone concentrations are associated with a high risk of breast cancer." *Ann Inter Med.* 1999; 130: 270–277.

Defay, R., et al. "Hormonal status and NIDDM in the European and Melanesia population of New Caledonia: a case-control study." *Inter Jour Obes Relet Metab Disord.* 1998; 22(9): The Caledonia DM (CALDIA) study Group, 927–934.

Dorgan, J., et al. "Serum sex hormone levels are related to breast cancer in postmenopausal women." *Environ Health Perspect.* 1997; 105(3): 583–585.

Kanaya, A., et al. "Glycemic effects of postmenopausal hormone therapy: the heart and estrogen/progestin replacement study." *Ann Intern Med.* 2003; 138(1): 1–9.

Mantzoros, C., et al. "Dehydroepiandrosterone sulfate and testosterone are independently associated with body fat distribution in premenopausal women." *Epidemiology.* 1996; 7(5): 513–515.

Nestler, J., et al. "Insulin as an effector of human ovarian and adrenal steroid metabolism." *Endocrinol Met Clincs North America.* 1991; 204: 807–823.

Nestler, J., et al. "Insulin inhibits adrenal 17-20-lyase activity in man." *J Clin Endocrinol Met.* 1992; 74(2): 362–367.

Schwarzbein, D. *The Schwarzbein Principle.* 1999; Deerfield Beach, FL: Health Communications, Inc., 225–226.

Schwarzbein, D. *The Schwarzbein Principle II.* 2002; Deerfield Beach, FL: Health Communications, Inc.

Smith, P. *What You Must Know About Vitamins, Minerals, Herbs, and More.* 2008; Garden City Park, NY: Square One Publishers.

Stoll, B. "Western nutrition and the insulin resistance syndrome: a link to breast cancer." *Eur Jour Clin Nutr.* 1999; 53(2): 83–87.

Tchernof, A., et al. "Obesity and metabolic complication contribution of dehydroepiandrosterone and other steroid hormones." *Jour Endocrinol.* 1996; 150(Supp 1): 155–164.

Toniolo, P., et al. "A prospective study of endogenous estrogens and breast cancer in postmenopausal women." *Jour Natl Cancer Inst.* 1995; 87(3): 190–197.

Vliet, E., et al. "New insights on hormones and mood." *Menopause Management*. 1993; June/July: 140–146, 154, 157.

## THYROID HORMONE

Adlin, V., et al. "Subclinical hypothyroidism: deciding when to treat." *Amer Fam Physician*. 1998; 57(4): 776–780.

Agid, O., et al. "Triiodothyronine augmentation of selective serotonin reuptake inhibitor in post traumatic stress disorder." *Jour Clin Psychiatry*. 2001; 62(3): 169–173.

Aksoy, I., et al. "Human liver dehydroepiandrosterone sulfatransferase: nature and extent of individual variation." *Clin Pharmacol Therapeutics*. 1993; 54(5): 498–506.

Arnold, L. "Alternative treatments for adults with attention-deficit hyperactivity disorder (ADHD)." *Ann NY Acad Sci*. 2001; 931: 310–341.

Barnes, B. *Hypothyroidism: The Unsuspected Illness*. 1976; New York: Harper and Row Publishers.

Beard, J., et al. "Impaired thermoregulation and thyroid function in iron deficiency anemia." *Am J Clin Nutr*. 1990; 52: 813–819.

Berger, N., et al. "Influence of selenium supplementation on the post-traumatic alterations of the thyroid axis: a placebo-controlled trial." *Intensive Care Med*. 2001; 27(1): 91–100.

Berry, M., et al. "The role of selenium in thyroid hormone action." *Endocrine Rev*. 1992; 13: 207–220.

Brownstein, D. *Iodine: Why You Need It, Why You Can't Live Without It*. 2004; West Bloomfield, MI: Medical Alternatives Press, 169.

Brownstein, D. *The Miracle of Natural Hormones*. 1998; West Bloomfield, Michigan: Medical Alternatives Press, 11.

Brownstein, D. *Overcoming Thyroid Disorders*. 2002; West Bloomfield, MI: Medical Alternatives Press, 8, 27, 37, 113.

Bunevicius, R., et al. "Effects of thyroxine as compared with thyroxine plus triiodothyroxine in patients with hypothyroidism." *NEJM*. 1999; Feb. 11: 424.

Cerillo, A., et al. "Free triiodothyronine: a novel predictor of postoperative atrial fibrillation." *Eur Jour Cardiothorac Surg*. 2003; 24(4): 487–492.

Christ-Crain, M., et al. "Elevated c-reactive protein and homocysteine values: cardiovascular risk factors in hypothyroidism? A cross-sectional and double-blind, placebo-controlled trial." *Atherosclerosis*. 2003; 166(2): 379–386.

DeGroot, L. *The Thyroid and Its Diseases*. 1996; New York: Churchill Livingstone, 342.

Divi, R., et al. "Anti-thyroid isoflavones from soybean: isolation, characterization, and mechanism of action." *Biochem Pharmacol*. 1997; 62(157): Fed Regester, 1087–1096.

Fernandez-Real, J., et al. "Thyroid function is intrinsically linked to insulin sensitivity and endothelium-dependent vasodilation in healthy euthyroid subjects." *Jour Clin Endocrin Med*. 2006; June 27.

Freake, H. "Iodine." In: *Stipanuk, M., ed. Biochemical and Physiological Aspects of Human Nutrition*. 2000; Philadelphia: WB Saunders, 761–781.

Friberg, L., et al. "Association between increased levels of reverse triiodothyronine and mortality after acute myocardial infarction." *Amer Jour Med*. 2001; 111(9): 699–703.

Ganapathy, S., et al. "Zinc, exercise, and thyroid hormone function." *Crit Rev Food Sci Nutr*. 1999; 39: 369–390.

Guyton, A. *A Textbook of Medical Physiology*. 2000; Philadelphia: WB Saunders.

Goldman, B. *Human Growth Factors*. 2003; Chicago: American Academy of Anti-Aging Physicians, 60.

Hak, A., et al. "Subclinical hypothyroidism is an independent risk factor for atherosclerosis and myocardial infarction in elderly women: The Rotterdam Study." *Ann Int Med*. 2000; 132(4): 270–278.

Hale, A., et al. "Subclinical hypothyroidism is an independent risk factor for atherosclerosis and MI in elderly women: The Rotterdam study." *Ann Inter Med*. 2000; 132: 270–278.

Hamilton, M., et al. "Safety and hemodynamic effects of IV triiodothyronine in advanced congestive heart failure." *Amer Jour Card*. 1998; 81(4): 443–447.

Hamilton, M., et al. "Thyroid hormonal abnormalities in heart failure: possibilities for therapy." *Thyroid*. 1996; 6(5): 527–529.

Hanaway, P. "Hormone essentials: Personalizing diagnosis and treatment." *Module I, Anti-Aging and Regenerative Medicine Fellowship*. 2007; Las Vegas, NV: Dec. 10–12.

Hertoghe, E. http://www.brodabarnes.org

Hertogue, J., et al. "Thyroid insufficiency. Is thyroxine the only valuable drug?" *Jour of Nutr & Environ Med*. 2001; 11: 159–166.

Hollowell, J., et al. *Jour of Clin Endo Met*. 2002; 87(2): 489–99.

Horst, C., et al. "Rapid stimulation of hepatic oxygen consumption by 3,5-di-iodo-1-thyrooninne." *Biochem J*. 1989; 261: 945–950.

Iervasi, G., et al. "Low T3 syndrome, a strong prognostic predictor of death in patients with heart disease." *Circulation*. 2003; 107: 708.

Kidd, P., et al. "ADHD in children: rationale for its integrative management." *Alt Med Rev*. 2000; 5(5): 402–428.

Kohrle, J. "The deiodinase family; selenoenzymes regulating thyroid hormone availability and action." *Cell Mol Life Sci*. 2000; 57: 1853–1863.

Lange, U., et al. "Thyroid disorders in female patients with ankylosing spondylitis." *Eur Jour Med Res*. 1999; 4(11): 468–474.

Lark, S. *The Menopause Self Help Book*. 1990; Berkeley, CA: Celestial Arts, 105.

Lenon, D., et al. "Diet and exercise training effects on resting metabolic rate." *Int J Obesity*. 1985; 9: 39–47.

Meinhold, H., et al. "Effects of selenium and iodine deficiency on iodothyronine deiodinases in brain, thyroid and peripheral tissue." *JAMA*. 1992; 19: 8–12.

Mendleson, J. "Alcohol effects on reproductive function in women." *Psychiatr Letter*. 1986; 4: 35–8.

Nedrebo, B., et al. "Plasma total homocysteine levels in hyperthyroid and hypothyroid patients." *Metabolism*. 1998; 47(1): 89–93.

Neeck, G., et al. "Neuroendocrine perturbations in fibromyalgia and chronic fatigue syndrome." *Rheum Dis Clin North Amer*. 2000; 26(4): 989–1002.

Nishida, M., et al. "Direct evidence for the presence of methylmercury bound in the thyroid and other organs obtained from mice give methylmercury; differentiation of free and bound methylmercuries in biological materials determined by volatility of methylmercury." *Chem Pharm Bull*. 1990; 38(5): 1412–1413.

Nishiyama, S., et al. "Zinc supplementation alters thyroid hormone metabolism in disabled patients with zinc deficiency." *J Am Coll Nut*. 1994; 13: 62–67.

Nishiyama, S., et al. "Zinc supplementation alters thyroid hormone metabolism in disabled patients with zinc deficiency." *Jour Amer Coll Nutr*. 1994; 13(1):62–67.

Pansini, F. "Effect of the hormonal contraception on serum reverse triiodothyronine levels." *Gynecol Obstet Invest*. 1987; 23: 133.

Rachman, B. "Managing endocrine imbalance; autoimmune-induced thyroidopathy and chronic fatigue syndrome." *Functional Medicine Approaches to Endocrine Disturbances of Aging*. 2001; Gig Harbor, WA: The Institute For Functional Medicine, 226.

Rea, W. *Chemical Sensitivity: Clinical Manifestations of Pollutant Overload. Volume III*. 1996; Boca Raton: CRC Press, Inc.

Rosenweig, P., et al. "Effect of iron supplementation on thyroid hormone levels and resting metabolic rate in two college female athletes: a case study." *Int Jour Sport Nutr Exerc Met*. 2000; 10: 434–443.

Rosenzweig, P., et al. "Iron, thermoregulation and metabolic rate." *Crit Rev Food Sci Nutr*. 1999; 39: 131–148.

Rouzier, N. "Thyroid replacement therapy." *Longevity and Preventive Medicine Symposium*. 2002; 2–4, 16.

Shimoyama, N., et al. "Serum thyroid hormone levels correlate with cardiac function and ventricular tachyarrhythmia in patients with chronic heart failure." *Jour Card*. 1993; 23(2): 205–213.

Starr, M. *Hypothyroidism, Type 2*. 2005; Columbia, MO: Mark Starr Trust.

Tagawa, N., et al. "Serum dehydroepiandrosterone, dehydroepiandrosterone sulfate, and pregnenolone sulfate concentrations in patients with hyperthyroidism and hypothyroidism." *Clinical Chem.* 2000; 46: 523–528.

Van den Beld, A. "Thyroid hormone concentrations, disease, physical function, and mortality in elderly men." *Jour of Clinic Endocrinology and Metabolism.* 2005; 90(12): 6403–6409.

Visser, T., et al. "Role of sulfation in thyroid hormone metabolism." *Chem Biol Interactions.* 1994; 92: 293–303.

Vliet, E. *Women Weight and Hormones.* 2001; New York: M. Evans & Company, 25, 127–128.

Vunevicious., B., et al. "Effects of thyroxine as compared with thyroxine plus triiodothyronine in patients with hypothyroidism." *NEJM.* 1999; 340: 424–429.

Wartofsky, L., et al. "The evidence for a narrower thyrotropin reference range is compelling." *Jour Clin Endo Met.* 2005; 90(9): 5483–5488.

Woeber, K. "Levothyroxine therapy and serum free thyroxine and free triiodothyronine concentrations." *Jour Endocrinol Invest.* 2002; 25(2):106–109.

## MELATONIN

Bland, J. "Obesity and endocrine signaling." *Improving Intercelluar Communication in Managing Chronic Illness.* 1999; Gig Harbor, Washington: Health Comm International, Inc., 124, 127.

Brzezinski, A., et al. "Melatonin in humans." *NEJM.* 1997; 336(3): 186–195.

Collins, J. *What's Your Menopause Type.* 2000; Roseville, CA: Prima Health, 239, 339.

Duell, P., et al. "Inhibition of LDL oxidation by melatonin requires supraphysiologic concentrations." *Clin Chem.* 1998; 44(9): 1931–1936.

Foss-Morgan, R. *Hormone Replacement Therapy.* 2000; Haddonfield, NJ: AntiAging and Longevity Medical Center of Haddonfield.

Lieberman, S. *The Real Vitamin and Mineral Book.* 1997; New York: Avery Publishing, 216–217.

Mills, E., et al. "Melatonin in the treatment of cancer: a systematic review of randomized controlled trials and meta-analysis." *Jour Pineal Res.* 2005; 39(4): 360–366.

Poeggeler, B., et al. "Melatonin a highly potent endogenous radical scavenger and electron donor: new aspects of the oxidation chemistry

of this indole accessed in vitro." *Ann NY Acad Sci.* 1994; 738: 419–421.

Reiter, R. "Melatonin: clinical relevance." *Best Pract Res Clin Endocrinol Metab.* 2003; 17(2): 273–285.

Reiter, R., et al. "Melatonin: reducing intracellular hostilities." *Endocrinologist.* 2004; 14(4): 222–228.

Sinatra, S. "Melatonin shows promise against age-related disorders." *Heart, Health and Nutrition.* 2007; 13(9): 6–7.

Tan, D., et al. "Melatonin: a potent endogeneous hydroxyl radical scavenger." *Endocrine J.* 1993; 1: 57–60.

Vliet, E., et al. "New insights on hormones and mood." *Menopause Management.* 1993; June/July: 140–146, 149–150.

## PROLACTIN

EMedicine. "Prolactin Deficiency." http://emedicine.medscape.com/article/124526-overview

Vliet, E. *Women Weight and Hormones.* 2001; New York: M. Evans & Company, 25, 49.

# PART II: AILMENTS AND PROBLEMS

## BLADDER PROBLEMS

Brocklehurst, J., et al. "Urinary infections and symptoms of dysuria in women aged 45-64 years: their relevance to similar findings in the elderly." *Age Ageing.* 1972; 1: 41-47.

Cardozo, L. "Role of estrogens in the treatment of female urinary incontinence." *Jour Amer Geriatr Soc.* 1990; 38: 326-330.

Elia, G., et al. "Estrogen effects on the urethra: beneficial effects in women with genuine stress incontinence." *Obstet Gynecol Sur.* 1993; 48: 509-513.

Jackson, S., et al. "The effect of oestrogen supplementation on post-menopausal urinary stress incontinence: a double-blind placebo-controlled trial." *Brit Jour Obstet Gynaecol.* 1999; 106(7): 711-718.

Vliet, E. "Hormone connections in urinary incontinence in women." *Top Ger Rehab.* 2000; 15(4): 16-30.

Vliet, E. *It's My Ovaries, Stupid.* 2003; New York : Scribner, 212, 231.

Vliet, E. "Menopause and perimenopause: the role of ovarian hormones in common neuroendocrine syndromes in primary care." *Primary Care Clinics in Office Practice.* 2002; 29: 43-67.

Yamanishi, T., et al. "Effect of functional continuous magnetic stimulation for urinary incontinence." *Jour Urology.* 2000; 163: 456-459.

## CANCER

American Cancer Society. "Cancer Facts and Figures 2006." http://www.cancer.org/downloads/STT/CAFF2006PWSecured.pdf.

American Cancer Society. "What are the risk factors for cervical cancer?" http://www.cancer.org/docroot/CRI/content/CRI_2_4_2X_What_are_the_risk_factors_for_cervical_cancer_8.asp.

Antinoro, L. "Curbing cancer's reach: little things that might make a big difference." *Environmental Nutrition.* 2006; 29(6):1, 4.

Augustin, L., et al. "Glycemic index and glycemic load in endometrial cancer." *Int Jour Cancer.* 2003; 105:404-407.

Becker, S., et al. "Expression of 25 hydroxyvitamin D3-lalpha-hydroxylase in human endometrial tissue." *Jour Steroid Biochem Mol Biol.* 2007; 103(3-5):771-775.

Berube, S., et al. "Vitamin D, calcium, and mammographic breast densities." *Cancer Epidemiol Bioimarkers Prev.* 2004; 9:466-472.

Boccardo, F. et al., "Serum enterolactone levels and the risk of breast cancer in women with palpable cysts." *Eur Jour Cancer.* 2004; 40(1):84-89.

Butterworth, C., et al. "Folate-induced regression of cervical intraepithelial neoplasia in users of oral contraceptive agents." *Amer Jour Clin Nutr.* 1980; 33:926.

Calle, E., et al., "Overweight, obesity, and mortality from cancer in a prospectively studied cohort of U.S. adults." *NEJM.* 2003; 348:1625-1638.

Cotran, R., et al. *Pathologic Basis of Disease.* 3rd ed. 1984; Philadelphia, Pennsylvania: W.B. Saunders.

Cui, X., et al. "Dietary patterns and breast cancer risk in the shanghai breast cancer study." *Cancer Epidemiol Biomarkers Prev.* 2007; 16(7):1443-1448.

Davis, S. "Night shift work, light at night, and risk of breast cancer." *Jour Natl Cancer Inst.* 2001; 93:1557-1562.

De Lyra, E., et al. "25(OH)D3 and 1,25(OH)D3 serum concentration and breast tissue expression of 1 alpha-hydroxylase, 24-hydroxylase and vitamin D receptor in women with and without breast cancer." *Jour Steroid Biochem Mol Biol.* 2006; 100(4-5):184-192.

Denkert, C., et al. "Expression of cyclooxygenase-2 is an independent prognostic factor in human ovarian carcinoma." *Amer Jour Path.* 2002; 160:893-903.

Dwivedi, C., et al. "Effect of calcium glucarate on beta-glucurondiase activity and glucarate content of certain vegetables and fruits." *Biochem Mol Metab Biol.* 1990; 43(2):83-92.

Fader, A. "Endometrial cancer and obesity: epidemiology, biomarkers, prevention, and survivorship." *Gynecol Oncol.* 2009 114(1):121-127.

Fallon, W. "Scientific methods to reduce breast cancer risk." *Life Extension Collector's Edition 2008.* 2008; p. 61-70.

Fimognari, C., et al. "Sulforaphane as a promising molecule for fighting cancer." *Mutat Res.* 2007; 635(2-3):90-104.

Folkers, K., et al. "Relevance of the biosynthesis of coenzyme Q-10 and of the four bases of DNA as a rationale for the molecular causes of cancer and a therapy." *Biochem Biophys Res Commun.* 1996; 224(2):358-361.

Folkers, K., et al. "Survival of cancer patients in therapy with coenzyme Q-10." *Biochem Biophysic Res Comm.* 1993; 1982, 241-245.

Franceschi, S. "The IARC commitment to cancer prevention: the example of papillomavirus and cervical cancer." *Recent Results Cancer Res.* 2005; 166:277-297.

Friedrich, M., et al. "Analysis of the vitamin D system in cervical carcinomas, breast cancer and ovarian cancer." *Recent Results Cancer Res.* 2003; 164:239-246.

Garland, C., et al. "Serum 25-hydroxyvitamin D and colon cancer: eight year prospective study." *Lancet*. 1989; 2(8673):1176-1178.

Garland, C., et al. "What is the dose-response relationship between vitamin D and cancer risk?" *Nutrition Rev*. 2007; 65(8):S91-S95.

Gnagnarella et al. "Glycemic index, glycemic load, and cancer risk: a meta-analysis." *American Jour of Clin Nutrition*. 2008; 87:1793-1801.

Greenlee, R., et al. "Cancer statistics." *CA Cancer Jour Clin*. 2001; 50:7-33.

Hardman, A., et al. "Physical activity and cancer risk." *Proc Nutr Soc*. 2001; 60(1):107-113.

Hemandez, B., et al. "Diet and high grade premaligant lesions of the cervix: evidence of a protective role of foliate, riboflavin, thiamin, and vitamin $B_{12}$." *Cancer Causes and Control*. 2003; 14(9):859-870.

Hilakivi-Clarke, L., et al. "Nutritional modulation of the cell cycle and breast cancer." *Endocr Relat Cancer*. 2004; 11(4):603-622.

Holick, M., et al. "Vitamin D deficiency." *NEJM*. 2007; 357(3):266-281.

Holick, M., et al. "Vitamin D: its role in cancer prevention and treatment." *Prog Biophys Mol Biol*. 2006; 92(1):49-59.

Imai, K., et al. "Personality types, lifestyle, and sensitivity to mental stress in association with NK activity." *Inter Jour Hyg Environ Health*. 2001; 204:67-73.

Imseis, R., et al. "Effect of calcitriol and pamidronate in multiple myeloma." *Amer Jour Med Sci*. 1999; 318(1):61-66.

Johnson, K. "Dairy products linked to ovarian cancer risk." *Family Practice News*. June 15, 2000: 8.

Kabut, G., et al. "Estrogen metabolism and breast cancer." *Epidemology*. 2006; 17(1):80-88.

Kim, H., et al. "Effects of naturally-occurring flavonoids and bioflavonoids on epidermal cyclooxygenase and lipoxygenase from guina pigs." *Prostagland Leuket Essent Fatty Acids*. 1998; 58:17-24.

Konety, B., et al. "Effects of vitamin D (calcitriol) on transitional cell carcinoma of the bladder in vitro and in vivo." *Jour Urol*. 2001; 165(1):253-258.

Krueger, C. "Cervical cancer: putting prevention into practice." *Townsend Letter*. April, 2009; 52-58.

La Vecchia, C., et al. "Monounsaturated and other types of fat, and the risk of breast cancer." *Eur Jour Cancer Prev*. 1998; 7:461-464.

Lajous, M., et al. "Glycemic load, glycemic index, and the risk of breast cancer among Mexican women." *Cancer Causes Control*. 2005; 16(10):1165-1169.

Lappe, J., et al. "Vitamin D and calcium supplementation reduces cancer risk: results of a randomized trial." *Amer Jour Clin Nutr*. 2007 85(6):1586-1591.

Larsson, S., et al. "Glycemic load, glycemic index and carbohydrate intake in relation to risk of stomach cancer. A prospective study." *Int Jour Cancer*. 2006; 1118:3167-3169.

Leitzmann, M., et al. "Prospective study of physical activity and risk of postmenopausal breast cancer." *Breast Cancer Res*. 2008.

Liang, Y., et al. "Suppression of inducible cyclooxygenase and inducible nitric oxide synthase by apigenin and related flavonoids in mouse macrophages." *Carcinogenesis*. 1999; 20:1945-1932.

Lieberman, S. *Glycemic Index Food Guide*. 2006; Garden City Park, NY: Square One Publishers.

Liu, X., et al. "Differential expression and regulation of cyclooxygenase-1 and 2- in two human breast cancer cell lines." *Cancer Res*. 1996; 56:5125-5127.

Malliard, V., et al. "N-3 and N-6 fatty acids in breast adipose tissue and related risk of breast cancer in a case-control study in Tours, France." *Inter Jour Cancer*. 2002; 98:78-83.

Mayo Clinic. "Ovarian Cancer." http://www.mayoclinic.com/health/ovarian-cancer/DS00293.

McCann, S., et al. "Dietary lignin intakes and risk of pre-and postmenopausal breast cancer." *Int Jour Cancer*. 2004; 111(3):440-443.

McCarl, M., et al. "Incidence of colorectal cancer in relation to glycemic index and load in a cohort of women." *Cancer Epidemiol Biomarkers Prev*. 2006; 15:892-896.

Michaud, D., et al. "Dietary glycemic load, carbohydrate, sugar, and colorectal cancer risk in men and women," *Cancer Epidemiol Biomarkers Prev.* 2005; 14:1138-1147.

Murray, M. *Encyclopedia of Nutritional Supplements.* 1996; Rocklin, California: Prima Publishing.

Murray, M. *How to Prevent and Treat Cancer with Natural Medicine.* 2002; New York, New York: Riverhead Books, 113.

National Cancer Institute. "Cervical cancer: screening—health professional information." http://health.yahoo.com/cervical cancer-diagnosis/cervical-cancer-screening-health-professional-informaton-nci-pdq/healthwise-nicdr 0000062756.html.

National Cancer Institute. "Endometrial Cancer." www.cancer.gov/cancerinfo/types/endometrial.

National Cancer Institute. "SEER Stat Fact Sheets." http://seer.cancer.gov/statfacts/html/ovary.html.

National Cancer Institute. "What you need to know about cancer of the cervix." National Institutes of Health Publication No. 08-2407. http://www.cancer.gov/cancertopics/wyntk/cervix.

O'Byrne, K., et al. "Chronic immune activation and inflammation as the cause of malignancy." *Brit Jour Cancer.* 2001; 85:473-483.

Peterlik, M. "Calcium, vitamin D and cancer." *Anticancer Res.* 2009; 29(9):3687-3698.

Polesel, J., et al. "Linoleic acid, vitamin D and other nutrient intakes in the risk of non-Hodgkin lymphoma: an Italian case-control study." *Ann Oncol.* 2006; 17(4):713-718.

Pung, A., et al. "Beta carotene and canthaxanthin inhibit chemically and physically-induced neoplastic transformation in 10T1/2 cells." *Carcinogenesis.* 1988; 9:1533-1539.

Purdie, D. "Epidemiology of endometrial cancer." *Best Pract Res Clin Obstet Gynecol.* 2002; 15(3):341-354.

Reichman, M., et al. "Effects of alcohol consumption on plasma and urinary hormone concentrations in premenopausal women," *Jour Natl Cancer Inst.* 1993; 85(9):692-693.

Sales, K., et al. "Cyclooxygenase-1 is up-regulated in cervical carcinomas: autocrine/paracrine regulation of cyclooxygenase-2. Prostaglandin e receptors, and angiogenic factors by cyclooxygenase-2." *Cancer Res.* 2002; 62:424-432.

Schernhammer, E., et al. "Rotating night shifts and risk of breast cancer in women participating in the Nurses' Health Study." *Jour Natl Cancer Inst.* 2001; 93:1563-1568.

Segerstrom, S. "Personality and the immune system: models, methods, and mechanisms." *Ann Behav Med.* 2000; 22:180-190.

Silvera, S., et al. "Dietary carbohydrates and breast cancer risk: A prospective study of the roles of oeverall glycemic index and glycemic load," *Int Jour Cancer.* 2005; 114:653-658.

Singletary, K., et al. "Alcohol and breast cancer: review of epidemiologic and experimental evidence and potential mechanisms." *JAMA.* 2001; 286:2143-2151.

Skinner, H., et al. "Vitamin D intake and the risk for pancreatic cancer in two cohort studies." *Cancer Epidemiol Biomarkers Prev.* 2006; 15(9):1688-1695.

Slattery, M., et al. "Dietary vitamin A, C, and E and selenium as risk factors for cervical cancer." *Epidemiol.* 1990; 1:8-15.

Tavani, A., et al. "Consumption of sweet foods and breast cancer risk in Italy," *Ann Oncol.* 2006; 17(2):341-345.

Theodoratou, E., et al. "Modification of the inverse association between dietary vitamin D intake and colorectal cancer risk by a Fok1 variant supports a chemoprotective action of vitamin D intake mediated through VDR binding." *Int Jour Cancer.* 2008; 23(9):2170-2179.

Thune, I., et al. "Physical activity and cancer risk: dose-response and cancer, all sites and site-specific." *Med Sci Sports Exerc.* 2001; 33(Suppl 6):530S-550S.

Tinelli, A. "Hormonal carcinogenesis and socio-biological development factors in endometrial cancer: a clinical review." *Acta Obstet Gynecol.* 2008; 87(11):1101-1113.

Van den Bemd, G., et al. "Vitamin D and vitamin D analogs in cancer treatment." *Curr Drug Targets.* 2002; 3(1):85-94.

Venkateswaran, V., et al.,"An understanding of low-carbohydrate, high-fat diets and cancer." *Seminars Prev Altern Med.* 2006; 2:136-140.

Walaszek, Z., et al. "Metabolism, uptake, and excretion of a D-glucaric acid salt and its potential use in cancer prevention." *Cancer Detect Prev.* 1997; 21(2):178-190.

Wright, J. "The 'unimportant' molecule curing cancer." *Townsend Letter.* April 2009, 66-70.

Yerby, C. "Coenzyme Q-10: new applications for cancer therapy." *Life Extensions.* Oct 2005; 50-56.

Zhang, X., et al. "Vitamin D receptor is a novel drug target for ovarian cancer treatment." *Curr Cancer Drug Targets.* 2006; 6(3):229-244.

## CERVICAL DYSPLASIA

Brinton, L. "Oral contraceptives and cervical neoplasia," *Contraception.* 1991; 43: 581–595.

Butterworth, C., et al. "Folate deficiency and cervical dysplasia," *JAMA.* 1992; 267: 528–533.

Butterworth, C., et al. "Improvement in cervical dysplasia associated with folic acid therapy in users of oral contraceptives." *Amer Jour Clin Nutr.* 1982; 35: 73–82.

Butterworth, C., et al. "Oral folic acid supplementation for cervical dysplasia. A clinical intervention trial." *Amer Jour Obstet Gynecol.* 1992; 166: 803–809.

Clarke, E., et al. "Smoking as a risk factor in cancer of the cervix: additional evidence from a case-control study." *Amer Jour Epidemiol.* 1982; 115: 59–66.

Dawson, E., et al. "Serum vitamin and selenium changes in cervical dysplasia" *Red Proc.* 1984; 43: 612.

De Vet, H., et al. "The effect of beta-carotene on the regression and progression of cervical dysplasia: a clinical experiment." *Jour Clin Epidermiol.* 1991; 44(3): 273–283.

De Vet, H., et al. "Risk factors for cervical dysplasia: implication for prevention." *Public Health.* 1994; 108: 241–249.

Giuliano, A., et al. "Antioxidant nutrients: associations with persistent human papillomavirus infection." *Cancer Epidemiol Biomark Prev.* 1997; 6: 917–923.

Goodman, M., et al. "Case-control study of plasma folate, homocysteine, vitamin $B_{12}$, and cysteine as markers of cervical dysplasia." *Cancer.* 2000; 89(2): 376–382.

Graham, V., et al. "Phase II trial of beta-all-trans-retinoic acid for cervical intraepithelial neoplasia delivered via a collagen sponge and cervical cap." *West Jour Med.* 1986; 145: 192–195.

Guillano, A., et al. "Can cervical dysplasia and cancer be prevented with nutrients?" *Nut Rev.* 1998; 5691: 9–16.

Harper, J., et al. "Erythrocyte folate levels, oral contraceptive use and abnormal cervical cytology." *Acta cytol.* 1994; 38: 324–330.

Hudson, T., et al. "Cervical Dysplasia." in Pizzorno, J., *Textbook of Natural Medicine 3rd Ed.* 2006; St. Louis, MS: Churchill Livingstone, 1572.

Hudson, T. "Menstrual cramps (dysmenorrheal): an alternative approach." *Townsend Newsletter.* Oct. 2006; 130–134.

Kwasnievska, A., et al. "Folate deficiency and cervical intraepithelial neoplasia," *Eur Jour Gynaecol Oncol.* 1997; 1896: 526–530.

La Vecchia, C., et al. "Dietary vitamin A and the risk of invasive cervical cancer," *Int Jour Cancer.* 1984; 34: 319–322.

Lindenbaum, J., et al. "Oral contraceptive hormones, folate, metabolism, and the cervical epithelium." *Amer Jour Clin Nutr.* 1975; 28(4): 346–353.

Liu, T., et al. "A longitudinal analysis of human papillomavirus 16 infection, nutritional status, and cervical dysplasia progression." *Cancer Epidemiol Biomarkers Prev.* 1995; 4: 373–380.

Lyon, J., et al. "Smoking and carcinoma in situ of the uterine cervix." *Amer Jour Public Health.* 1983; 73: 558–562.

Mackeras, D., et al. "Randomized double-blind trial of beta-carotene and vitamin C in women with minor cervical abnormalities." *Brit Jour Cancer.* 1999; 79(9–10): 1448–1453.

Manetta, A., et al. "Beta-carotene treatment of cervical intraepitheial neoplasia: a phase II study." *Cancer Epidemiol Biomarkers Prev.* 1996; 5(11): 929–932.

Meyskens, F., et al. "Enhancement of regression of cervical intraepithelial neoplasia II (moderate dysplasia) with topically applied all-trans-retinoic acid: a randomized trial." *Jour Natl Cancer Inst.* 1994; 86: 539–543.

Nagata, C., et al. "Serum carotenoids and vitamins and risk of cervical dysplasia from a case-control study in Japan." *Brit Jour Cancer.* 1999; 81(7): 1234–1237.

Nagata, C., et al. "Serum retinol level and risk of subsequent cervical cancer in cases with cervical dysplasia." *Cancer Invest.* 1999; 17(4): 253–258.

Orr, J., et al. "Nutritional status of patients with untreated cervical cancer, II. Vitamin assessment." *Amer Jour Obstet Gynecol.* 1985; 151: 632–635.

Pelleter, O. "Vitamin C and tobacco." *Int Jour Vitam Nutr Res.* 1977; 16: 147–169.

Pelton, R. *The Nutritional Cost of Drugs.* 2004; Englewood, CO: Morton Publishing Company, 69.

Peng, Y., et al. "Concentrations of carotenoids, tocopherols, and retinol in paired plasma and cervical tissue of patients with cervical cancer, precancer, and noncancerous diseases." *Cancer Epidemiol Biomarkers Prev.* 1998; 7(4): 347–350.

Piyathilake, C., et al. "Folate is associated with the natural history of high-risk human papillomaviruses." *Cancer Res.* 2004; 64: 8788–8793.

Ramaswamy, P., et al. "Vitamin $B_6$ status in patients with cancer of the uterine cervix." *Nutr Cancer.* 1984; 6: 176–180.

Robbins, S., et al. *Pathologic Basis of Disease, 3rd Ed.* 1984; Philadelphia, PA: WB Saunders, 1123–1138.

Romney, S., et al. "Effects of beta-carotene and other factors on outcome of cervical dysplasia and human papillomavirus infection." *Gynecol Oncol.* 1997; 65(3): 483–492.

Romney, S., et al. "Nutrients antioxidants in the pathogenesis and prevention of cervical dysplasias and cancer." *Jour Cell Biochem.* 1995; 23(Suppl): 96–103.

Romney, S., et al. "Plasma vitamin C and uterine cervical dysplasia." *Amer Jour Obstet Gynecol.* 85; 151: 978–980.

Romney, S., et al. "Retinoids and the prevention of cervical dysplasias," *Amer Jour Obstet Gynecol.* 1981; 141:890–894.

Sedjo, R., et al. "Effect of plasma micronutrients on clearance of oncogenic human papillomavirus (HPV) infection (United States)." *Cancer Causes Control.* 2003; 14: 319–326.

Sedjo, R., et al. "Human papillomavirus persistence and nutrients involved in the methylation pathway among a cohort of young women." *Cancer Epidemiol Biomarkers Rev.* 2002; 11(4): 353–359.

Smith, P. *What You Must Know About Vitamins, Minerals, Herbs & More.* 2008; Garden City Park, NY: Square One Publishers, 240–241.

Streiff, R. "Folate deficiency and oral contraceptives." *JAMA.* 1970; 214: 105–08.

Thomson, S., et al. "Correlates of total plasma homocysteine: folic acid, copper, and cervical dysplasia." *Nutrition.* 2000; 16(6): 411–416.

Ursin, G., et al. "Oral contraceptive use and adenocarcinoma of the cervix." *Lancet.* 1994; 344: 1390–1394.

Van Eenwyk, J., et al., "Dietary and serum carotenoids and cervical intraepithelial neoplasia." *Inter Jour Cancer.* 1991; 48(1): 34–38.

Van Eenwyk, J., et al. "Folate, vitamin C, and intraepithelial neoplasia." *Cancer Epidemiol Biomarkers Prev.* 1992; 1(2): 119–124.

Wassertheil-Smoller, S., et al. "Dietary vitamin C and uterine cervical dysplasia." *Amer Jour Epidemiol.* 1981; 114: 714–724.

Werbach, M. "Cervical dysplasia." *Townsend Newsletter.* 2006; Nov.: 143–144.

Whitehead, N., et al. "Megaloblastic changes in the cervical epithelium: association with oral contraceptive therapy and reversal with folic acid." *JAMA.* 1973; 226: 1421–1424.

Wylie-Rosett, J., et al. "Influence of vitamin A on cervical dysplasia and carcinoma in situ." *Nutr Cancer.* 1984; 6: 49–57.

## CYSTIC ACNE

Vliet, E. *It's My Ovaries, Stupid.* 2003; New York: Scribner, 212, 231.

## DES BABIES

Mayo Clinic. "Vaginitis." http://www.mayo clinic.com/health/vaginitis/DS00255

United States Department of Health and Human Services Centers for Disease Control and Prevention. "DES Daughters." http://www.cdc.gov/DES/consumers/daughters/index.html

Vliet, E. *It's My Ovaries, Stupid.* 2003; NY: Scribner, 103.

## ENDOMETRIOSIS

Alexander, M., et al. "Oral beta-carotene can increase the number of okT4+cells in human blood." *Immunol Lett.* 1985: 9: 221–224.

Anderson, R. "The immunostimulatory, anti-inflammatory and anti-allergic properties of ascorbate." *Adv Nutr Res.* 1984; 6: 19–45.

Biskind, M., et al. "Effect of B complex deficiency on inactivation of estrone in the liver." *Endocrinology.* 1942; 31: 109–114.

Butler, E., et al. "Vitamin E in the treatment of primary dysmenorrheal." *Lancet.* 1955; 1: 844–847.

Cobelis, L., et al. "High plasma concentrations of di-(2-ethylhexyl)-phthalate in women with endometriosis." *Human Repro.* 2003; 18(7):1512--1515.

Decapite, L. "Histology, anatomy and antibiotic properties of Vitex agnus castus." *Ann Facul Agr Univ Studi Perugia.* 1967; 22: 109–126.

Flower, A., et al. "Seeking an oracle: using the Delphi process to develop practice guidelines for the treatment of endometriosis with Chinese herbal medicine." *Jour Altern Complement Med.* 2007; 13(9): 969–976.

Foyouzi, N., et al. "Effects of oxidants and antioxidants on proliferation of endometrial stromal cells." *Fertil Steril.* 2004; 82, Suppl 3: 1019–1022.

Goldin, B., et al. "Effect of diet on excretion of estrogens in pre- and postmenopausal women." *Cancer Res.* 1981; 41: 3771–3773.

Grodstein, F., et al. "Relation of female infertility to consumption of caffeinated beverages." *Amer Jour Epid.* 1993; 137: 1353–1360.

Grodstein, F., et al. "Relation of female infertility to consumption of caffeinated beverages." *Amer Jour Epidemiol.* 1993; 137: 1353–1360.

Hadfield, R., et al. "Linkage and association studies of the relationship between endometriosis and genes encoding the detoxification enzymes GSTM1, GSTT1, and CYP1A1." *Mol Hum Repro.* 2001; 7(11):1073–1078.

Hanaway, P. "Hormone essentials: Personalizing diagnosis and treatment." *Module I, Anti-Aging and Regenerative Medicine Fellowship.* 2007; Dec. 10–12: Las Vegas, NV.

Hellier, J., et al. "Organochlorines and endometriosis." *Chemosphere.* 2008; 71(2): 203–210.

Hudson, T. "Chronic pelvic pain: part II management with natural medicine." *Townsend Letter.* 2006; Dec: 148–155.

Hudson, T. "Endometriosis." *Pizzorno, J., Textbook of Natural Medicine 3rd Ed.* 2006.

Igarashi, S., et al. "Endometeriosis and free radicals." *Gynecol Obstet Invest.* 1999; 48: 29–35.

Kappas, A., et al. "Nutrition-endocrine interactions: induction of reciprocal changes in the delta 4–5 alpha-reduction of testosterone and the cytochrome P-450-dependent oxidation of estradiol by dietary macronutrients in man." *Pro Natl Acad Sci USA.* 1983; 80: 7646–7649.

Leibovitz, B., et al. "Bioflavonoids and polyphenols: medical applications." *Jour Opt Nutr.* 1993; 2: 17–35.

London, R., et al. "Endocrine parameters and alpha-tocopherol therapy of patients with mammary dysplasia." *Cancer Res.* 1981; 41: 3811–3813.

Louis, M.S.: *Churchill Livingstone.* 1643–1648.

Marchese, M. "Endometriosis." *Townsend Letter.* April 2009, 59–62.

Mayani, A., et al. "Dioxin concentrations in women with endometriosis." *Human Reproduction.* 1997; 12: 373–375.

Mayo Clinic. "Endometriosis." http://www.mayoclinic.com/health/endometriosis/DS00289/DSECTION=causes

Michnovicz, J., et al. "Altered estrogen metabolism and excretion in humans following consumption of indole-3-carbinol." *Nutr Cancer.* 1991; 16: 59–66.

Murphy A., et al. "Endometriosis: a disease of oxidative stress?" *Semin Repro Endocrinol.* 1998; 16(4): 263–273.

Parazzini, F., et al. "Selected food intake and risk of endometriosis." *Hum Reprod.* 2004; 19(8): 1755–1759.

Podgaec, S., et al. "Endometriosis: an inflammatory disease with a Th2 immune response component." *Hum Reprod.* 2007; 22(5): 1373–1379.

Querleu, D. "Treatment of rectovaginal endometriosis." *Presse Med.* 1997; 26(16): 774–777.

Spallholz, J., et al. "Immunologic response of mice fed diets supplemented with selenite selenium." *Proc Sox Exp Biol Med.* 1973; 143: 685–689.

Tanaka, T. "A novel anti-dysmenorrhea therapy with cyclic administration of two Japanese herbal medicines." *Clin Exp Obstet Gynecol.* 2003; 30(2–3): 95–98.

Tremblay, L. "Reproductive toxins conference—pollution prevention network." *Endometriosis Assoc Newsl.* 1996; 17: 13–15.

Watson, R., et al. "Effect of beta-carotene on lymphocyte subpopulations in elderly humans: evidence for a dose-response relationship." *Amer Jour Clin Nutr.* 1991; 53: 90–94.

Wieser, F., et al. "Evolution of medical treatment for endometriosis: back to the roots?" *Hum Reprod Update.* 2007; 13(5): 487–499.

## FIBROCYSTIC BREAST DISEASE

University of Maryland Medical Center. "Fibrocystic breast disease - Symptom." http://www.umm.edu/ency/article/000912sym.htm

## FIBROIDS

Crayhon, R. "Aging well in the 21st century." Seminar. 2002; Detroit, MI.

Goldberg, B. "Fibroids an alternative approach." *Townsend Letter for Doctors and Patients.* Jan 2000; 84–96.

Hudson, T. "Uterine fibroids: an alternative approach." *Townsend Letter for Doctors and Patients.* May 2000; 153–157.

## HEART DISEASE

Ballantyne, C.M.; Vasudevan, A.R. "Cardiometabolic risk assessment: An approach to the prevention of cardiovascular disease and diabetes mellitus." *Clinical Cornerstone.* 2005; 7(2/3): 7–17.

Barnebei, V., et al. "Plasma homocysteine in women taking hormone replacement therapy: the postmenopausal estrogen/progestin intervention (PEPI) trial." *J Women's Health Gend Based Med.*1999; 8(9):1167–1172.

Berger, J.S.; Roncaglioni, M.C.; Avanzini, F; et al. "Aspirin for the primary prevention of cardiovascular events in women and men: A sex-specific meta-analysis of randomized controlled trials." *JAMA.* 2006; 295(3): 306–313.

Bladbjerg, E.M.; Skouby, S.O.; Anderson, L.F.; Jespersen, J. "Effects of different progestin regimes in hormone replacement therapy on blood coagulation factor VII and tissue factor pathway inhibitor." *Human Reproduction.* 2002; 17(12): 3235–41.

Boudoulas, K.D.; Cooke, G.E.; Roos, C.M. "The polymorphism of glycoprotein IIIa functions as a modifier for the effect of estrogen on platelet aggregation." *Arch Pathol Lab Med.* 2001; 125(1): 112–115.

Boushey, C., et al. "A quantitative assessment of plasma homocysteine as a risk factor for vascular disease. Probably benefits of increasing folic acid intake." *JAMA.* 1995; 274: 1949–1957.

Braunstein, J.B.; Kershner, D.W.; Bray, P.; et al. "Interaction of hemostatic genetics with hormone therapy." *Chest.* 2002; 121: 906–920.

Carmel, R., et al. "Hormone replacement therapy and cobalamin status in elderly women." *Am J Clin Nutr.* 1996: 64(6): 856–859.

Clarke, R, et al. "Underestimation of the importance of homocysteine as a risk factor for cardiovascular disease in epidemiological studies." *J Cardiovasc Risk.* 2001; 8(6): 363–369.

Cortellaro, M.; Boschett, C.; Cofrnacesco, E.; et al. "The PLAT study: hemostatic function in relation to atherothrombotic ischemic events in vascular disease patients; principal results." *Arterioscler Thromb.* 1992; 12: 1063–1070.

Crandall, C; Palla, S.; Reboussin. B.; et al. "Cross-sectional association between markers of inflammation and serum sex steroid levels in the PEPI trial." *J Womens Health.* 2006; 15(1): 14–23.

DeCree, C., et al. "Influence of exercise and menstrual cycle phase on plasma homocysteine levels in young women prospective study." *Scand J Med Sci Sports.* 1999; 9(5): 272–278.

Dubey, K.; Tofovic, S.; Jackson, E. "Cardiovascular pharmacology of estradiol metabolites." *Journal of Pharmacology and Experimental Therapeutics.* 2004; 308: 403–409.

Eskandari, F.; Mistry, S.; Martinez. P.; et al. "Younger, premenopausal women with major depressive disorder have more abdominal fat and increased serum levels of prothrombotic factors: implications for greater cardiovascular risk." *Metabolism Clinical and Experimental.* 2005; 54: 918–924.

Esparza, J.; Fox, C.; Harper, I.T.; et al. "Daily energy expenditure in Mexican and USA Pima Indians: low physical activity as a possible cause of obesity." *Int J Obes Relat Metab Disord.* 2000; 24(1): 55–59.

Espeland, M., et al. "Effect of postmenopausal hormone therapy on lipoprotein (a) concentration PEPI investigators, postmenopausal estrogen/progestin interventions." *Circulation.* 1998; 97(10): 979–986.

Fonseca, V.A. "The metabolic syndrome, hyperlipidemia, and insulin resistance." *Clinical Cornerstone.* 2005; 7(2/3): 61–72.

Ford, E., et al. "Does exercise reduce inflammation? Physical activity and c-reactive protein among U.S. adults." *Epidemiology.* 2002; 13(5): 561–568.

Ford, E., et al. "Homocysteine and cardiovascular disease: a systemic review of the evidence with special emphasis on case-control studies and nested case-control studies." *Int J Epidemiol.* 2002; 31(1): 59–70.

Garcia-Moll, X.; Zouridakis, E.; Cole, D.; Kaski, J.C. "C-reactive protein in patients with chronic stable angina: Differences in baseline serum concentration between women and men." *European Heart Journal.* 2000; 21: 1598–1606.

Gierach, G.L.; Johnson, B.D.; Merz, N.B.; Kelsey, S.F; et al. "Hypertension, menopause, and coronary artery disease risk in the women's ischemia syndrome evaluation (WISE) study." *J of the Am Col Cardio.* 2006; 47: 50S-58S.

Grancha, S.; Estelles, A.; Tormo, G.; et al. "Plasminogen activator inhibitor-1 (PAI-1) promoter 4G/5G genotype and increased PAI-1 circulating levels in postmenopausal women with coronary artery disease." *Thromb Haemost.* 1991; 81(4): 516–21.

Grundy, S.M. "A constellation of complications: The metabolic syndrome." *Clinical Cornerstone.* 2005; 7(2/3): 36–45.

Hackam, D., et al. "What level of plasma homocysteine should be treated? Effects of vitamin therapy on progression of carotid atherosclerosis in patients with homocysteine levels above and below 14 micromol/L." *Amer Jour Hypertens.* 2000; 13: 105–110.

Hak A., et al. "Increased plasma homocystine after menopause." *Atherosclerosis.* 2000; 149(1): 163–168.

Hoffman, C.J.; Miller, R.H.; Lawson, W.E.; et al. "Elevation of factor VII activity and mass in young adults at risk of ischemic heart disease." *J Am Coll Cardiol.* 1989; 14: 941–946.

Homocysteine Lowering Trialists' Collaboration. "Dose-dependent effects of folic acid on blood concentrations of homocysteine: a meta-analysis of the randomized trials." *Amer Jour Clin Nutr.* 2005; 82(4): 80–112.

Houston, M. "Treatment of Insulin Resistance, The Metabolic Syndrome and Type II Diabetes: Part 2. Overview of Nutrition, Nutraceuticals, Antioxidants, Supplements, Vitamins, Minerals, Exercise, Weight Management and Lifestyle Changes." *Fellowship in Anti-Aging and Functional Medicine.* 2007.

Hu, P.; Greendale, G.A.; Palla, S.L.; Reboussin, B.A.; et al. "The effects on hormone therapy on the markers of inflammation and endothelial function and plasma matrix metalloproteinase-9 level in postmenopausal women: The postmenopausal estrogen progestin intervention trial." *Atherosclerosis.* 2006; 185: 347–352.

Jacobsen, S.; Buch, P.; Rasmussen, J.; et al. "Most NSAIDS rise risk of death after heart attack." *Abstract 1838*. 2005; Dallas, TX: American Heart Association Annual Conference.

Jespersen, J.; Munkvad, S.; Gram, J.B. "The fibrinolysis and coagulations systems in ischemic heart disease: risk markers and their relation to metabolic dysfunction of the arterial intima." *Don Med Bull*. 1993; 40(4): 495–502.

Jialal, I., et al. "Inflammation and atherosclerosis: the value of the high-sensitivity c-reactive protein assay as a risk marker." *Am J Clin Pathol*. 2001; 116 (Suppl):S108–S115.

Kelly, G. "Folates: supplemental forms and therapeutic applications." *Alern Med Rev*. 1998; 3(3): 208–220.

Kip, K.E.; Marroquin, O.C.; Shaw, L.F.; et al. "Global inflammation predicts cardiovascular risk in women: A report from the Women's Ischemia Syndrome Evaluation (WISE) study." *Am Heart J*. 2005; 150(5): 900–906.

Kroom, U.B.; Silfverstolpe, G.; Tengborn, L. "The effects of transdermal estradoil and oral conjugated estrogens on haemostasis variables." *Thrombosis and Haemostasis*. 1994; 71(4): 420–3.

Laszlo, B.; Tanko, Y.; Bagger, G. "Enlarged waist combined with elevated triglycerides is a strong predictor of accelerated atherogenesis and related cardiovascular mortality in postmenopausal women." *Circulation*. 2006; 111: 1883–1890.

Lavoie, K.L.; Miller, S.B.; et al. "Anger, negative emotion, and cardiovascular reactivity during interpersonal conflict in women." *J Psychosom Res*. 2001; 51(3): 503–512.

Loscaizo, J., et al. "Lipoprotein (a): a unique risk factor for atherothrombotic disease." *Arterlosclerosis*. 1990; 10(5): 672–679.

Madsen, T., et al. "C-reactive protein, dietary n-3 fatty acids, and the extent of coronary artery disease." *Am J Cardiol*. 2001; 88(10): 1139–1142.

Mallnow, M., et al. "Homocysteine, diet and cardiovascular disease: a statement for health-care professionals from the Nutrition Committee, American Heart Association." *Circulation*. 1999; 99: 178–182.

Matsumoto, Y., et al. "High level of lipoprotein (a) is a strong predictor for progression of coronary artery disease." *J Atharoscler Thromb*. 1998; 5(2): 47–53.

Mayo Clinic. "Heart Disease." http://www.mayoclinic.com/health/heart-disease/DS01120

McCully, K. "Homocysteine and the heart revolution." *Disorders of Intercellular Mediators and Messengers, Their Relationship to Functional Illness*. 1999; Gig Harbor, Washington: The Functional Medicine Institute, 87.

Minshall, R.; Miyagawa, K.; Chadwick, C.; et al. "In vitro modulation of primate coronary vascular muscle cell reactivity by ovarian steroid hormones." *The FASEB Journal*. 1998; 12: 1419–1429.

Miyagawa, K.; Rosch, J.; Stanczyk, F.; et al. "Medroxyprogesterone interferes with ovarian steroid protection against coronary vasospasm." *Nature Medicine*. 1997; (3); 3: 324–327.

Molloy, A., et al. "Thermolabile variant of 5,10-methylenetetrahydrofolate reductase associated with low red-cell folates: implications for folate intake recommendations." *Lancet*. 1997; 349: 1591–1593.

Morrison, J.; Friedman, L.; Harlan, W.; Harlan, L.; et al. "Development of the metabolic syndrome in black and white adolescent girls: a longitudinal assessment." *PEDIATRICS*. 2005; 116: 1178–1182.

Nappo, F., et al. "Impairment of endothelial function by acute hyperhomocysteinemia and reversal by antioxidant vitamins." *JAMA*. 1999; 281: 2113–2118.

Nash, D.T. "C-Reactive protein: A promising new marker of cardiovascular risk?" *Consultant*. 2005; 453–460.

Nesta, R.W. "Managing cardiovascular risk in patients with metabolic syndrome." *Clinical Cornerstone*. 2005; 7(2/3): 46–51.

Nourhashemi, F., et al. "Alzheimer's disease: protective factors." *Am J Clin Nutr*. 2000; 71(2): S643–S649.

Onzer, M. "VAP cholesterol testing: advanced technology uncovers hidden cardiovascular risks." *Life Extension*. 2007; May: 67–71.

Patel, C.; Edgerton, L.; Flake, D. "What precautions should we use with statins for women of childbearing age?" *The Journal of Family Practice.* 2006; 55(1): 75–77.

Pletcher, M.; Baron, R. "Primary prevention of cardiovascular disease in women: new guidelines and emerging strategies." *Advanced Studies in Medicine.* 2005; 5: 412–419.

Psaty, B.M.; Smith, N.L.; Menaitre, R.N.; et al. "Hormone replacement therapy, prothrombotic mutations, and the risk of incident nonfatal myocardial infractions in postmenopausal women." *JAMA.* 2001; 285(7): 906–913.

Quyyumi, A.A. "Women and ischemic heart disease: Pathophysiologic implications from the WISE study and future research steps." *J of the Am Coll of Cardio.* 2006; 47: 66S-71S.

Rao, L.V.; Pendurthi, U.R. "Tissue factor-factor VIIa signaling." *Arterioscler Thromb Vasc Biol.* 2005 Jan; 25(1): 47–56.

Refsum, H., et al. "Homocysteine and cardiovascular disease." *Ann Rev Med.* 1998; 49: 31–62.

Reuben, D.B.; Palla, S.L.; Reboussin, B.A.; Crandall, C.; et al. "Progestins affect mechanism of estrogen-induced C-reactive protein stimulation." *The American Journal of Medicine.* 2006; 119: 167–168.

Ridker, P., et al. "Novel risk factors for systemic atherosclerosis: a comparison of C-reactive protein, fibrinogen, homocysteine, lipoprotein (a) and standard cholesterol screening as predictors of peripheral arterial disease." *JAMA.* 2001; 285(19): 2481–2485.

Ridker, P.M.; Hennekens, C.H.; Rifai, N; et al. "Hormone replacement therapy and increased plasma concentration of C-reactive protein." *Circulation.* 1999; 100: 713–716.

Ridker, P.M.; Buring, J.E.; Shih, J.; et al. "Prospective study of C-reactive protein and the risk of future cardiovascular events among apparently healthy women." *Circulation.* 1998; 98: 731–733.

Rifai, N.; Buring, J.E.; I-Min, Lee.; et al. "Is C-Reactive protein specific for vascular disease in women?" *Annals of Internal Medicine.* 2002; 136(7): 529–533.

Rodriguez, I.; Kilborn, M.J.; Liu X.X.; et al. "Drug-induced QT prolongation in women during the menstrual cycle." *JAMA.* 2001; 285: 1322–1326.

Rost, N., et al. "Plasma concentration of C-reactive protein and risk of ischemic stroke and transient ischemic attack: the Framingham study." *Stroke.* 2001; 32(11): 2575–2579.

Roussouw, J.E. "Hormones, genetic factors, and gender differences in cardiovascular disease." *Cardiovascular Research.* 2002; 53: 550–557.

Sader, M.A.; Celermajer, D.S. "Endothelial function, vascular reactivity and gender differences in the cardiovascular system." *Cardiovascular Reasearch.* 2002; 53: 597–604.

Scarbabin, P.; Oger, E.; Plu-Bureau, G. "Differential association of oral and transdermal oestrogen-replacement therapy with venous thromboembolism risk." *The Lancet.* 2003; 362: 428–32.

Shaw, L.J.; Merz, N.B.; Pepine, C.J.; Reis, S.E.; et al. "Insights from the NHLBI-sponsored women's ischemia syndrome evaluation (WISE) study." *J of the Am Coll Cardio.* 2006; 47: 4S-29S.

Sinatra, S. *Heart, Health & Nutrition Newsletter.* 2007; July: 2–3.

Sinatra, S. *Heart Sense for Women.* 2000; Washington D.C.: LifeLine Press, 53–55, 62–64, 66, 68–69, 108.

Steptoe, A.; Lundwall, K.; Cropley, M. "Gender, family structure and cardiovascular activity during the working day and evening." *Soc Sci Med.* 2000; 50(4): 531–539.

Stern, L., et al. "Conversion of 5-formyltetrahydrofolic acid to 5-methyltetrahydrofolic acid is unimpaired in folate-adequate persons homozygous for the C677T mutation in the methylenetetrahydrofolate reductase gene." *Jour Nutr.* 2000; 30(9): 2238–2242.

Stoney C., et al. "Plasma homocysteine levels increase in women during psychological stress." *Life Sci.* 1999; 64(25): 2359–2365.

Stork, S.; Baumann, K.; Von Schacky, C.; Angerer. "The effect of 17 beta estradiol on MCP-1 serum levels in postmenopausal women." *Cardiovascular Research.* 2002; 53: 643–649.

Straczek, C.; Oger, E.; Beau Yon de Jonage-Canonico, M.; et al. "Prothrombotic mutations, hormone therapy, and venous thromboembolism among postmenopausal women: Impact of the route of estrogen administration." *Circulation*. 2005; 112: 3495–3500.

Superko, H. "Did grandma give you heart disease? The new battle against coronary artery disease." *Amer Jour Cardiol*. 1998; 82(9A): 34Q– 46Q.

Tallova, J., et al. "Changes of plasma total homocysteine levels during the menstrual cycle." *Eur J Clin Invest*. 1999; 29(12): 1041–1044.

*Third Report of the National Cholesterol Education Program (NCEP) Expert Panel on Detection, Evaluation, and Treatment of High Blood Cholesterol in Adults. (Adult Treatment Panel III) Final Report*. 2002; Washington, DC: NIH Publication: No. 02–5215.

Toprak, A., et al. "The effect of postmenopausal hormone therapy with or without folic acid supplementation on serum homocysteine level." *Climacteric*. 2005; 8(3): 279–286.

Toth, P.P. "C-reactive protein: a new tool for evaluating cardiovascular disease risk.3." *Family Practice Recertification*. 27(4)L 27–39.

Tsai, J., et al. "Promotion of vascular smooth muscle cell growth by homocysteine: a link to atherosclerosis." *Proc Natl Acad Sci USA*. 1994; 91: 6369–6373.

Ueland, P., et al. "The controversy over homocysteine and cardiovascular risk." *Amer Jour Clin Nour*. 2000; 72: 324–332.

Van Baal, W., et al. "Cardiovascular disease risk and hormone replacement therapy (HRT). A review based on randomized, controlled studies in postmenopausal women." *Curr Med Chem*. 2000; 7(5): 499–517.

Van Baal, W.; Kenemans, P.; Van der Mooren, M.J.; et al. "Increased C-reactive protein levels during short-term hormone replacement therapy in healthy postmenopausal women." *Thrombosis and Haemostasis*. 1999; 81(6): 925–8.

Vagnini, F. *The Side Effects Bible*. 2005; NY: Broadway Books, 67–70.

Verhoef, P., et al. "Plasma total homocysteine, B vitamins and risk of coronary atherosclerosis." *Arterioscler Thromb Vasc Biol*. 1997; 17: 989–995.

Vinik, A.I. "The metabolic basis of atherogenic dyslipidemia." *Clinical Cornerstone*. 2005;7 (2/3): 27–35.

Vourilainen, S., et al. "Enhanced in vivo lipid peroxidation at elevated plasma total homocysteine levels." *Arterioscler Thomb Vasc Biol*. 1999; 19:1263–1266.

Walsh, J.M.E.; Pignone, M. "Drug treatment of hyperlipidemia in women." *JAMA*. 2004; 291: 2243–2252.

Wise, D.E.; Dewester J. "Metabolic syndrome and associated cardiovascular disease risk." *Am Acad Fam Physicians*. 2004: CME Bulletin 3(2): 1–5.

Wittstein, I.S.; Thiemann, D.R.; Lima, J.A.C.; et al. "Neurohumoral features of myocardial stunning due to sudden emotional stress." *NEJM*. 2005; 352(6): 539–48.

Wright, D.; Poller, L.; Thomson, J.M.; et al. "The effect of hormone replacement therapy on the age-related rise of factor VIIc, and its activity state." *Thrombosis Research*. 1997; 85(6): 455–464.

Yaffe, K.; Kanaya, A.; Lindquist, K.; et al. "The metabolic syndrome, inflammation, and risk of cognitive decline." *JAMA*. 2004; 292: 2237–2242.

## HORMONES AND SKIN

Aslam, M., et al. "Pomegranate as a cosmeceutical source: pomegranate fractions promote proliferation and procollagen synthesis and inhibit matrix metalloproteinase-1 production in human skin cells." *Jour Ethnopharmacol*. 2006; 103(3): 311–318.

Blatt, T. "Stimulation of skin's energy metabolism provides multiple benefits for mature human skin." *Biofactor*. 2005; 25(1–4): 179–185.

Goldfaden, G. "Protecting hands against unsightly aging." *Life Extension*. May 2007; 87–90.

Greco, M., et al. "Marked aging-related decline in efficiency of oxidative phosphorylation in human skin fibroblasts." *FASEB Jour*. 2003; 17(12):1706–1708.

Manuskiatti, W., et al. "Hyaluronic acid and skin: wound healing and aging." *Int Jour Dermatol*. 1996; 35(8): 539–544.

Passi, S., et al. "The combined use of oral and topical lipophilic antioxidants increases their levels both in sebum and stratum corneum." *Biofactors*. 2003; 18(1–4): 289–297.

Sander, C., et al. "Photoaging is associated with protein oxidation in human skin in vivi," *Jour Invest Dermatol*. 2002; 118(4): 618–625.

Saral, Y., et al. "Protective effects of topical alpha-tocopherol acetate on UVB irradiation in guinea pigs: importance of free radicals." *Physiol Res*. 2002; 51(3): 285–290.

Shippen, E. *Testosterone Syndrome*. 1998; New York: M. Evans & Company Inc., 145, 150.

Uhoda, I., et al. "Split face study on the cutaneous tensile effectiveness of 2-dimethylaminoethanol (deanol) gel." *Skin Res Technol*. 2002; 893: 164–167.

Weindl, G., et al. "Hyaluronic acid in the treatment and prevention of skin diseases: molecular biological, pharmaceutical, and clinical aspects." *Skin Pharmacol Physiol*. 2004; 17(5): 207–213.

Whiteman, D., et al. "Determinants of melanocyte density in adult human skin." *Arch Dermatol Res*. 1999; 291(9): 511–556.

## MENOPAUSE

Abramson, J. *Overdosed America*. 2004; New York, New York: HarperCollins.

Alexander, K.P.; Chen, A.Y.; Roe, M.T.; et al. "Excess dosing of antiplatelet and antithrombin agents in the treatment of Non-ST-Segment elevation Acute coronary Syndrome." *JAMA*. 2005; 294: 3108–3116.

Bower, A.D.; Burkett, G.L. "Family physicians and generic drugs: a study of recognition, information sources, prescribing attitudes, and practices." *Journal of Family Practice*. 1987; 24: 612–616.

Caudill, T.S.; Johnson, M.S.; Rich, E.C.; McKinney, P. "Physicians, pharmaceutical sales representatives and the cost of prescribing." *Archives of Family Medicine*. 1996; 5: 201–206.

Chew, L.D., et al. "A Physician Survey of the Effect of Drug Sample Availability on Physician' Behavior." *Journal of General Internal Medicine*. 2000; 15: 478–483.

Croasdale, M. "Innovative funding opens new residency slots." *American Medical News*. 2006; 49(4): 1–4.

Cutler, W. *Hysterectomy: Before and After*. 1988; NY: Harper & Row, 27.

Decision Resources, Inc. "PCPs More Influenced by Aggressive Marketing of Bipolar Drugs than Psychiatrists." http://pharma licensing.com/public/press/view/113515628 3_43a91c3b93429/ pcps-more-influenced-by-aggressive-marketing-of-bipolar-drugs-than-psychiatrists

Dieperink, M.E.; Drogemuller, L. "Industry-sponsored grand rounds and prescribing behavior." *Journal of the American Medicinal Association*. 2000; 285: 1443–1444.

Glenmullen, J. *Prozac Backlash: Overcoming the Dangers of Prozac, Zoloft, Paxil, and Other Antidepressants with Safe, Effective Alternatives*. 2000; New York: Simon and Schuster.

Hanley, J. "Female Empowerment in the decisions from PMS to menopause." *Functional Medicine Approaches to Endocrine Disturbances of Aging*. 2001; Gig Harbor, Washington: The Functional Medicine Institute, 12.

Kassirer, J.P. "Why should we swallow what these studies say?" *Advanced Studies in Medicine*. 2004; 4(8): 397–398.

Kravitz, R.; Epstein, R.; Feldman, M.; et al. "Influence of patients' requests for direct-to-consumer advertised antidepresants." *JAMA*. 2005; 293(16): 1995–2002.

Laux, M. *Natural Woman, Natural Menopause*. 1997; New York: HarperCollins, 20, 99.

Lexchin, J. "Doctors and detailers: therapeutic education or pharmaceutical promotion?" *Int J Health Services*. 1989; 19: 663–679.

Lurie, N.; et al. "Pharmaceutical representitives in academic medical centers: interaction with faculty and housestaff." *Journal of General Internal Medicine*. 1990; 5: 240–243.

Majumdar, S.R.; Almasi, E.A.; Stafford, R.S. "Promotion and prescribing of hormone therapy after report of harm by the Women's Health Initiative." *JAMA*. 2004; 292: 1983–1988.

Mayo Clinic. "Menopause." http://www.mayo clinic.com/health/menopause/DS00119/ DSECTION=risk-factors

Murray, M. *The Healing Power of Herbs*. 1995; CA: Prima Publications, 375.

Nachtigall, L. *Estrogen The Facts Can Change Your Life*. 1995; New York: HarperCollins, 27, 66.

O-Reilly, K.B. "AMA opt-out program will keep prescribing data from drug reps." *American Medical News*. 2006; 49(20): 1–2.

Orlowski, J.P.; Wateska, L. "The effects of pharmaceutical firm enticements on physician prescribing patterns: There's no such thing as a free lunch." *Chest*. 1992; 102: 270–273.

Schmidt, L.M.; Gotzsche, P.C. "Of mites and med: references bias in narrative review articles: a systematic review." *The Journal of Family Practice*. 2005; 54(4): 334–338.

Stephenson, K.; Jones, B.; Stephenson, D. "The role of drug promotion in hormone replacement therapy prescribing in the United States." *International Journal of Pharmaceutical Compounding*. 2006; 10(3): 174–181.

Vliet, E., *It's My Ovaries, Stupid!* 2003; New York: Scribner, 60–61.

Vliet, E. "New insights on hormones and mood." *Menopause Management*. 1993; June/July: 140–146.

Vliet, E. *Women Weight and Hormones*. 2001; New York: M. Evans & Company, 25, 35, 39–40, 107.

Welch Cline, R.J.; Young, H.N. "Direct-to-consumer print ads for drugs: So they undermine the physician-patient relationship?" *The Journal of Family Practice*. 2005; 54(12): 1049–1052.

## MIGRAINES

Vliet, E. "An approach to perimenopausal migraine." Menopause Management. 1995; 4(6): 25-33.

Vliet, E. *It's My Ovaries, Stupid*. 2003; New York: Scribner, 212, 231.

## OSTEOPOROSIS

Berkner, K. "The physiology of vitamin K nutriture and vitamin K-dependent protein function in atherosclerosis." *Jour Throm Haemost*. 2004; 2(2): 2118–2132.

Bland, J. *Clinical Nutrition: A Functional Approach*. 1999; Gig Harbor, WA: Institute for Functional Medicine, 147, 163–164, 166, 179.

Bland, J. "Nutrients as Biological Response Modifiers." *Applying Functional Medicine in Clinical Practice*. 2002; Gig Harbor, WA: Functional Medicine Institute, 35.

Bonjour, J, et al. "Nutritional aspects of hip fractures." *Bone*. 1996; 18(3Suppl):S13–S44.

Booth, S., e al. "Effects of a hydrogenated form of vitamin K on bone formation and resorption." *Amer Jour Clin Nutr*. 2001; 74(6): 783–790.

Chetkowski, R., et al. "Biologic effects of transdermal estradiol." *NEJM*. 1986; 314: 1615–1620.

Colgan, M. *The New Nutrition*. 1995; Vancover: Apple Publishing, 63–64, 91, 101–104, 148–149.

Collins, J. *What's Your Menopause Type*. 2000; Roseville, CA: Prima Health, 189.

Crook, D. "The metabolic consequences of treating postmenopausal women with non-oral hormone replacement therapy." *Brit Jour Obstet Gynaecol*. 1997; 104(Suppl 16): S4–S13.

Crook, T. *The Memory Cure*. 1998; NY: Pocket Books, 159.

Demer, L., et al. "Novel mechanisms in accelerated vascular calcification in renal disease patients." *Curr Opin Nephrol Hyperten*. 2002; 11(4): 437–433.

Erenus, M., et al. "Comparison of effects of continuous combined transdermal with oral estrogen and oral progestogen replacement therapies on serum lipoproteins and compliance." *Climacteric*. 2001; 4: 228–234.

Fillion, M. *Natural Prostate Healers*. 1999; Paramus, NJ: Prentice Hall Press, 90.

Flore, C., et al. "Response of biochemical markers of bone turnover to estrogen treatment in post-menopausal women: evidence against an early anabolic effect on bone formation." *J Endocrinol Invest*. 2001; 24: 423–509.

Gaby, A., *Nutritional Therapy in Medical Practice*. 2003; Carlisle, PA: Nutrition Seminars, 33.

Gelejinse, J. et al. "Dietary intake of menaquinone is associated with a reduced risk of coronary heart disease: the Rotterdam Study." *Jour Nutr*. 2004; 134(11): 3100–3105.

Germano, R. *The Osteoporosis Solution*. 1999; New York: Kensington Publishing Corp., 99, 101–103.

Gilson, G., et al. "A perspective on HRT for women: Picking up the pieces after the Women's Health Initiative Trial, Part 1." *Intern Jour of Pharmaceutical Compounding*. 2003; 7(4): 250–256.

Gittleman, A. *Super Nutrition For Menopause*. 1998; New York: Avery Publishing, 52–53, 61, 79, 104.

Goepp, J. "Vitamin K's delicate balancing at." *Life Extension*. 2006; April: 59–67.

Greenblatt, R., et al. "The fate of a large bolus of exogenous estrogen administered to postmenopausal women." *Maturitas*. 1979; 2: 29–35.

Head, K. "Estriol: Safety and efficacy." *Altern Med Rev*. 1998; 3: 101–113.

Hesley, R., et al. "Monitoring estrogen replacement therapy and identifying rapid bone loses with an immunoessay for deoxypyridinoline." *Osteoporosis Int*. 1998; 8(2): 159–164.

Holick, M., et al. "Calcium and vitamin D. Diagnostics and therapeutics." *Clin Lab Med*. 2000; 20(3): 569–590.

Hunt, C., et al. "Dietary boron modifies the effects of vitamin D3 nutrition on indices of energy substrate utilization and mineral metabolism in the chick." *J Bone Miner Res*. 1994; 9(2): 171–182.

Iwamoto, J., et al. "Combined treatment with $K_2$ and bisphosphonate in postmenopausal women with osteoporosis." *Yonsei Med Jour*. 2003; 4495: 751–756.

Kaneki, M., et al. "Vitamin $K_2$ as a protector of bone health and beyond." *Clin Calcium*. 2005; 15(4): 605–610.

Koh, K., et al. "Effects of hormone replacement therapy on fibrinolysis in postmenopausal women." *NEJM*. 1997; 336: 683–690.

Laux, M. *Natural Woman, Natural Menopause*. 1997; New York: HarperCollins, 20, 34, 51.

Lieberman, S. *The Real Vitamin and Mineral Book*. 1997; New York: Avery Publishing, 85, 165, 216.

Manonai, J., et al. "Effect of oral estriol on urogenital symptoms, vaginal cytology, and plasma hormone level in postmenopausal women." *Jour Med Assoc Thai*. 2001; 84: 539–544.

Marie, P., et al. "Mechanisms of action and therapeutic potential of strontium in bone." *Calcif Tissue It*. 2001; 69(3): 121–129.

Meunier, P., et al. "The effects of strontium ranelate on the risk of vertebral fracture in women with postmenopausal osteoporosis." *NEJM*. 2004; 350: 459–468.

Meunier, P., et al. "Strontium ranelate: dose-dependent effects in established postmenopausal vertebral osteoporosis—a 2-year randomized placebo controlled trial." *Jour Clin Endocrinol Metab*. 2002; 87(5): 2060–2066.

Miggiano, G., et al. "Vitamin K and diet: problems and prospects." *Clin Ther*. 2005; 156(1–2): 41–46.

Nachtigall, L. *Estrogen The Facts Can Change Your Life*. 1995; New York: HarperCollins, 27, 154, 156.

Nachtigall, L., et al. "Serum estradiol-binding profiles in postmenopausal women undergoing three common estrogen replacement therapies: Associations with sex hormone-binding globulin, estradiol, estrone levels." *Menopause*. 2000; 7: 243–250.

Nguyen, U., et al. "Aspartame ingestion increases urinary calcium, but not oxalate excretion, in healthy subjects." *Jour Clin Endocrinol Metab*. 1998; 83(1): 165–168.

O'Donnell, S., et al. *Cochrane Database Syst Rev*. 2006; 18(4): CD005326.

Okano, T. "Vitamin D, K and bone mineral density." *Clin Calcium*. 2005; 15(9): 1489–1494.

Prior, J., et al. "Progesterone as a bone trophic hormone." *Endocrine Reviews*. 1990; 11: 386–398.

Reese, A., et al. "Low-dose vitamin K to augment anticoagulation control." *Pharmacotherapy*. 2005; 25(12): 1746–1751.

Reginster, J., et al. "Prevention of early postmenopausal bone loss by strontium ranelate: he randomized, two-year, double-masked, dose-ranging. placebo-controlled REVOS trial." *Osteoporosis Int*. 2002; 13(12): 94–131.

Reginster, J., et al. "Strontium ranelate reduces fractures in osteoporotic women." *Jour Clin Endocrinol Metab*. 2005; 90(5): 2816–2822.

Richards, J., et al. "Effects of selective serotonin reuptake inhibitors on the risk of fracture." *Arch Inter Med*. 2007; 167(2): 188–194.

Ryan-Harshman, M., et al. "Bone health. New role for vitamin K?" *Can Fam Physician.* 2004; 50: 993–997.

Scarabin, P., et al. "Effects of oral and transdermal estrogen/progesterone regimens on blood coagulation and fibrinolysis in postmenopausal women. A randomized controlled trial." *Arterioscler Thromb Vasc Biol.* 1997; 17: 3071–3078.

Shoji, S., et al. "Vitamin K and vascular calcification." *Clin Calcium.* 2002; 12(8): 1123–1128.

Sinatra, S. *Heart Sense for Women.* 2000; Washington D.C.: LifeLine Press, 108, 164.

Sowers, M. "A prospective study of bone mineral content and fracture in communities with differential fluoride exposure." *Am J Epidemiol.* 1991; 133(7): 649–660.

Stevenson, M., et al. *Health Technol Assess.* 2007; 11(4): 1–134.

Takahashi, K., et al. "Safety and efficacy of oestriol for symptoms of natural or surgically induced menopause." *Hum Repro.* 2000; 15: 1028–1036.

Taylor, M. "Unconventional estrogens: Estriol, biest, and triest." *Clin Obstet Gynecol.* 2001; 44: 864–879.

Ushiroyama, T., et al. "Estrogen replacement therapy in postmenopausal women: A study of the efficacy of estriol and changes in plasma gonadotropin levels." *Gynecol Endocrinol.* 2001; 15: 74–80.

Vasquez, A., et al. "The clinical importance of vitamin D (cholecalciferol): a paradigm shift with implications for all healthcare providers." *Alternative Therapies.* 2004; 10(5): 28–36.

Vehkavaara, S., et al. "Effects of oral and transdermal estrogen replacement therapy on markers of coagulation, fibrinolysis, inflammation and serum lipids and lipoproteins in postmenopausal women." *Throm Haemost.* 2001; 85: 619–625.

Weber, P. "The role of vitamins in the prevention of osteoporosis—a brief status report." *Int Jour Vitamin Nutr Res.* 1999; 69(3): 194–197.

Wilkin, T., et al. "Changing perceptions in osteoporosis." *Br Med J.* 1999; 318: 862–865.

Yang, Y., et al. "Long-term proton pump inhibitor therapy and risk of hip fracture." *JAMA.* 2006; 296(24): 2947–2953.

## PCOS

Ahene, S., et al. "Polycystic ovary syndrome." *Nurs Stand.* 2004; 18(26): 40–44.

Atimo, W., et al. "Familial associations in women with polycystic ovary syndrome." *Fertil Steril.* 2003; 80(1): 143–145.

Barnea, E., et al. "Stress-related reproductive failure." *Jour IVF Embryo Transfer.* 1991; 8: 15–23.

Carey, A., et al. "Evidence for a single gene effect causing polycystic ovaries and male pattern baldness." *Clin Endocrinol.* 1993; 38(6): 653–658.

De Leo, V., et al. "Polycystic ovary syndrome and type 2 diabetes mellitus." *Minera Ginecol.* 2004; 56(1): 53–62.

Falola, E., et al. "Body composition, fat distribution and metabolic characteristics in lean and obese women with polycystic ovary syndrome." *Jour Endocrinol Invest.* 2004; 27(5): 424–429.

Gambineria, A., et al. "Obesity and the polycystic ovary syndrome." *Int Jour Obes Relat Metab Disord.* 2002; 26(7): 883–896.

Gonzalez, C., et al. "Polycystic ovarian disease: clinical and biochemical expression." *Ginecol Obstet Mex.* 2003; 71: 253–258.

Gonzalez, C., et al. "Polycystic ovaries in childhood: a common finding in daughters of PCOS patients. A pilot study." *Hum Repro.* 2002; 17(3): 771–776.

Harris, C. and Cheung, T. *The PCOS Protection Plan.* 2006; Carlsbad, CA: Hay House Inc.

Legro, R., et al. "Prevalence and predictors of risk for Type 2 diabetes mellitus and impaired glucose tolerance in polycystic ovary syndrome: a prospective, controlled study in 254 affected women." *Jour Clin Endocrinol Metabol.* 1999; 84(1): 165–169.

Kocak, M., et al. "Metformin therapy improves ovulatory rates, cervical scores, and pregnancy rates in clomiphene citrate-resistance women with polycystic ovary syndrome." *Fertil and Steril.* 2002; 77(1): 101–106.

Marantides, D., et al. "Management of polycystic ovary syndrome." *Nurse Pract.* 1997;
22(12): 34–38, 40–41.

Mayo Clinic. "Polycystic Ovary Syndrome."
http://www.mayoclinic.com/health/polycys-
tic-ovary-syndrome/DS00423/DSECTION=
tests-and-diagnosis

Morin-Papunen, L., et al. "Metformin therapy
improves the menstrual pattern with minimal
endocrine and metabolic effects in women
with polycystic ovary syndrome." *Fertil Steril.*
1998; 69(4): 691–696.

Pelusi, B., et al. "Type 2 diabetes and the polycystic ovary syndrome." *Minerva Ginecol.* 2004;
56(1): 41–51.

Robinson, S., et al. "Postprandial thermogenesis is reduced in polycystic ovary syndrome
and is associated with increased insulin resistance." *Clin Endocrinol.* 1992; 36(6): 537–543.

Smith, P. *Vitamins: Hype or Hope.* 2004; Traverse
City, Michigan: Healthy Living Books, 210–211.

Solomon, C., et al. "Long or irregular menstrual cycle as a marker for the risk of type
2 diabetes mellitus." *JAMA.* 2001; 286(19):
2421–2426.

Strauss, J., et al. "Some new thoughts on the
pathophysiology and genetics of polycystic
ovary syndrome." *Ann NY Aci Sci.* 2003; 997:
42–48.

Tsilchorozidou, T., et al. "Altered cortisol
metabolism in polycystic ovary syndrome:
insulin enhances 5 alpha-reduction but not
the elevated adrenal steroid production
rates." *Jour Clin Endocrino Metab.* 2003;
88(12): 5907– 5913.

Urbanek, M., et al. "Thirty-seven candidate
genes for PCOS: Strongest evidence of linkage
is follistatin." *Proc Nat Acd Aci.* 1999; 38(6):
653–658.

Vandermolen, D., et al. "Metformin increases
the ovultory rate and pregnancy rate from
clomiphene citrate in patients with polycystic
ovary syndrome who are resistant to
clomiphene citrate alone." *Fertil Steril.* 2001;
75(2): 310–315.

WebMD. "Polycystic Ovary Syndrome (PCOS)
- Topic Overview." http://women.webmd.
com/tc/polycystic-ovary-syndrome-pcos-
topic-overview?page=3

## POSTPARTUM DEPRESSION

Ahokas, A., et al. "Sublingual oestrogen treatment of postnatal depression." *Lancet.* 1998;
351(9096): 109–112.

Baird, D., et al. "Cigarette smoking associated
with delayed conception." *JAMA.* 1985; 253:
2979.

Becker, U., et al. "Menstrual disturbances and
fertility in chronic alcoholic women." *Drug and
Alcohol Dependence.* 1989; 24 :75–82.

Bloch, M., et al. "Effects of gonadal steroids in
women with a history of postpartum depression." *Amer Jour Psychiatry.* 2000; 157(6): 924–930.

Chen, E., et al. "Exercise and reproductive
dysfunction." *Fertil Steril.* 1999; 71(1): 1–6.

Cooper, G., et al. "Follicle-stimulating hormone concentrations in relation to active and
passive smoking." *Obstet Gynecol.* 1996; 85: 407.

Cooper, R., et al. "Endocrine disruptors and reproductive development: a weight of evidence
overview." *Jour Endocrinol.* 1997; 152: 159.

Feely, M., et al. "Health risks to infants from
exposure to PCBs, PCDDS, and PCDFs." *Food
Addit Contam.* 2000; 17(4): 325–333.

Ferraroni, M., et al. "Alcohol consumption and
risk of breast cancer: a multicenter Italian case-
control study." *European Jour of Cancer.* 1998;
34: 1403–1409.

Freeman, M. "Omega-3-fatty acids and perinatal depression: a review of the literature and
recommendations for future research."
*Prostaglandins Leukot Essential Fatty Acids.*
2006; 75(4–5): 291–297.

Gregoire, A., et al. "Transdermal oestrogen for
treatment of severe postnatal depression."
*Lancet.* 1996; 347: 930–933.

Henderson, A., et al., "The treatment of severe
postnatal depression with oestradiol skin
patches," *Lancet.* 1991; 338:816.

Hirata, J., et al. "Does dong quai have estrogenic effects in postmenopausal women? A
double-blind, placebo-controlled trial." *Fertil
Steril.* 1997; 68: 981–986.

Holladay, S. "Prenatal immunotoxicant exposure and postnatal autoimmune disease." *Environ Health Perspect.* 1999; 107 (Suppl 5):
68887–68891.

Mattison, D., et al. "The effect of smoking on oogenesis, fertilization, and implantation." *Semin Repro Endocrinol.* 1989; 7: 219.

Mattison, D., et al. "Reproductive toxicity: male and female reproductive systems as targets for chemical injury." *Med Clin North Amer.* 1990; 74: 391.

Mayo Clinic. "Postpartum Depression." http://www.mayoclinic.com/health/postpartum-depression/DS00546/DSECTION=risk-factors

Mendelson, J., et al. "Acute alcohol effects on plasma estradiol levels in women." *Psychopharmacology.* 1988; 94: 464–467.

Nagata, C., et al. "Decreased serum estradiol concentration associated with high dietary intake of soy products in premenopausal Japanese women." *Nutrition and Cancer.* 1997; 29(3): 228–233.

Pirke, K., et al. "Dieting influences the menstrual cycle: vegetarian versus nonvegetarian diet." *Fertility and Sterility.* 1968; 45(6): 1083–1088.

Rees, A., et al. "Role of omega-3-fatty acids as a treatment for depression in the perinatal period." *Aust NZ Jour Psychiatry.* 2005; 39(4): 274–280.

Sharara, F., et al. "Environmental toxicants and female reproduction." *Fertility Steril.* 1998; 70(4):613–622.

Smith, E., et al. "Occupational exposures and risk of female infertility." *Jour Occup Environ Med.* 1997; 39: 138.

Thomas, R., et al. "Thyroid disease and reproductive function: a review." *Obstet Gynecol.* 1987; 70: 789–798.

Valimaki, N., et al. "Acute effects of alcohol on female sex hormones." *Alcohol Clin Exp Res.* 1983; 7:289–293.

Van Voorhis, B., et al. "Effects of smoking on ovulation induction for assisted reproductive techniques." *Fertil Steril.* 1992; 58: 981.

Vliet, E. *It's My Ovaries, Stupid.* 2003; New York: Scribner, 108–120, 272.

Von Borstel, R. "Metabolic and physiologic effects of sweeteners." *Clin Nutr.* 1985; 4(6):215–20.

Whitten, P., et al. "Potential adverse effects of phytoestrogens." *Jour of Nutrition.* 1995; 125 (Suppl): S776.

Yeh, J., et al. "Effects of smoking on steroid production, metabolism, and estrogen-related diseases." *Semin Repro Endocrinol.* 1989; 7: 326.

## POD AND POF

Anaasti, J. "Premature ovarian failure: an update." *Fertility and Sterility.* 1998; 70(1): 1–15.

Berga, S. "Stress and ovarian function." *Amer Jour Sports Med.* 1996; 24(6Suppl): S36–S37.

Bullen, B., et al. "Endurance training effects on plasma hormonal responsiveness and sex hormone excretion." *Jour Appl Phys Respirat Environ Exercise Physiol.* 1984; 56(6): 1453–1463.

Coulam, C. "Premature gonadal failure." *Fertility and Sterility.* 1982; 38: 645–650.

Dionyssiou-Asteriou, A., et al. "Variations of serum hormone levels in young exercising women." *Clin Endocrinol.* 1999; 51(2): 258–260.

Gloor, H. "Autoimmune oophoritis." *Amer Jour Clin Path.* 1984; 81: 105–109.

Harrison, R., et al. "Ovarian impairments of female recreational distance runners during a season of training." *Annals of Human Biology.* 1998; 25(4): 345–357.

Hoek, A., et al. "Premature ovarian failure and ovarian autoimmunity." *Endocrinology Rev.* 1997; 18(1): 1077–1134.

Kim, J., et al. "Autoimmune ovarian failure." *Brit Jour Obstetrics and Gynaecology.* 1995; 21: 59–66.

Leer, M., et al. "Secondary amenorrhea due to autoimmune ovarian failure." *Australian and New Zealand Jour Obstet and Gynecol.* 1988; 158: 1–5.

Locke, R., et al. "Exercise and primary dysmenorrhoea." *Brit Jour Sports Med.* 1999; 33(4): 227.

Mayo Clinic. "Premature Ovarian Failure." http://www.mayoclinic.com/health/premature-ovarian-failure/DS00843/DSECTION=symptoms

Muechler, E., et al. "Autoimmunity in premature ovarian failure." *International Jour Fertility.* 1991; 36(2): 99–103.

Vliet, E. *It's My Ovaries, Stupid.* 2003; NY: Scribner, 6.

Wheatcroft, N., et al. "Is subclinical ovarian failure an autoimmune disease?" *Human Reproduction.* 1997; 12: 244–249.

Williams, D., et al. "Premenopausal cytomegalovirus oophritis." *Histopathology.* 1990; 16: 405–407.

Williams, N., et al. "Effects of short-term strenuous exercise upon corpus luteum function." *Med Sci Spors Exerc.* 1999; 31(7): 949–958.

## PMDD

Mayo Clinic. "What is premenstrual dysphoric disorder (PMDD)? How is it treated?" http://www.mayoclinic.com/health/pmdd/AN01372

## PREMENSTRUAL SYNDROME (PMS)

Butler, E., et al. "Vitamin E in the treatment of primary dysmenorrhoea." *Lancet.* 1955; 1: 844–847.

Chuong, C., et al. "Zinc and copper levels in premenstrual syndrome." *Fertil Steril.* 1994; 62: 313–320.

Costello, C., et al. "Estrogenic substances from plants. I. Glycyrrhiza." *Jour Amer Pharm Soc.* 1950; 39: 177–180.

Dittmar, F. "Premenstrual syndrome. Treatment with a phytopharmaceutical." *Therapiewoche Gynakol.* 1992; 5: 60–68.

Farese, R., et al. "Licorice-induced hypermineralcorticoidism." *NEJM.*1991; 325: 1223–1227.

Halbreich, U., et al. "The prevalence, impairment, impact, and burden of premenstrual dysphoric disorder (PMS/PMDD)." *Psychoneuroendocrinology.* 2003; 28 (Suppl 3): 1–23.

Harada, M., et al. "Effect of Japanese angelica root and peony root on uterine contraction in the rabbit in situ." *Jour Pharmacobiodyn.* 1984; 7: 304–311.

Harel, L., et al. "Supplementation with omega-3-polyunsaturated fatty acids in the management of dysmenorrhea in adolescents." *Amer Jour Obstet Gynecol.*1996; 174(4): 1335–1338.

Harlow, S., et al. "A longitudinal study of risk factors for the occurrence, duration, and severity of menstrual cramps in a cohort of college women." *Brit Jour Obstet Gynecol.* 1996; 103: 1134–1142.

Hudgins, A. "Niacin for dysmenorrheal." *Amer Pract and Digest of Treat.* 1952; 3: 892–893.

Hudgins, A. "Vitamins P, C, and niacin for dysmenorrhea therapy." *Western Jour Surgery and Gynecol.* 1954; 62: 610–611.

Hudson, T. "Chronic pelvic pain: Part II management with natural medicine." *Townsend Letter.* 2006; Dec.: 148–155.

Hudson, T. "Menstrual cramps (dysmenorrheal): an alternative approach." *Townsend Newsletter.* 2006; Oct.: 130–134.

Hudson, T., et al. "Premenstrual Syndrome." in Pizzorno, J., *Textbook of Natural Medicine 3rd Ed.* 2006; St. Louis, MS: Churchill Livingstone, 2053–2065.

Hyman, M. "The life cycles of women: restoring balance." *Alternative Therapies.* 2007; 13(3): 10–16.

Kohama, T., et al. "Analgesic efficacy of French maritime pine bark extract in dysmenorrhea: an open clinical trial." *Reprod Med.* 2004; 49(10): 828–832.

Kumagai, A., et al. "Effect of glycyrrhizin on estrogen action." *Endocrinol Japon.* 1967; 14: 34–38.

Mayo Clinic. "Menstrual Cramps." http://www.mayoclinic.com/health/menstrual-cramps/DS00506

Mayo Clinic. "Premenstrual Syndrome (PMS)." http://www.mayoclinic.com/health/premenstrual-syndrome/DS00134/DSECTION=symptoms

MSNBC. "The Menstrual Cycle." http://www.msnbc.com/news/wld/graphics/menstrual_cycle_dw2.swf

Peteres-Welte, C., et al. "Menstrual abnormalities and PMS. Vitex agnus-castus." *Therapiewoche Gynakol.* 1994; 7: 49–52.

Pickles, V., et al. "Prostaglandins in endometrium and menstrual fluid from normal dysmenorrheic subjects." *Brit Jour Obstet Gynecol.* 1965; 72: 185.

Pickles, V., et al. "Prostaglandins in the human endometrium." *Int Jour Fertil.* 1967; 12: 335.

Rosner, W., et al. "Sex hormone-binding globulin mediates steroid hormone signal transduction at the plasma membrane." *Jour Steroid Biochem Mol Biol.* 1999; 69(1–6): 481–485.

Schellenberg, R. "Treatment for the premenstrual syndrome with agnus castus fruit extract: prospective, randomized, placebo controlled study." *BMJ*. 2001; 322: 134–137.

Schildge, E. "Essay on the treatment of premenstrual and menopausal mood swings and depressive states." *Rigelh Biol Umsch*. 1964; 19: 18–22.

Stevinson, C., et al. "A pilot study of Hypericum perforatum for the treatment of premenstrual syndrome." *BJOG*. 2000; 107; 870–876.

Stormer, F., et al. "Glycyrrhizic acid in liquorice—evaluation of health hazard." *Fed Chem Toxicol*. 1993; 31: 303–312.

Tamborini, A., et al. "Value of standardized Ginkgo biloba extract in the management of congestive symptoms of premenstrual syndrome." *Jour Rev Fr Gynecol Obstet*. 1993; 88: 447–457.

Tseng, Y., et al. "Rose tea for relief of primary dysmenorrhea in adolescents: a randomized controlled trial in Taiwan." *Jour Midwifery, Womens Health*. 2005; 50(5): 51–57.

## Vulvodynia

Vliet, E. *It's My Ovaries, Stupid*. 2003; New York : Scribner, 212, 231.

Vliet, E. "Menopause and perimenopause: the role of ovarian hormones in common neuroendocrine syndromes in primary care." *Primary Care Clinics in Office Practice*. 2002; 29: 43-67.

## PART III: HORMONE REPLACEMENT THERAPY

## What is HRT?

Abrahamsen, B.; Nommevie-Nielsen, B.; et al. "Cytokines and bone loss in a 5 year longitudinal study-hormone replacement therapy suppresses serum soluble interleukin-6 receptor and increases interleukin-1-receptor antagonist: the Danish Osteoporosis Prevention Study." *J of Bone and Mineral Reasearch*. 2000; 15(8): 1545–54.

Ahlgrimm, M. *The HRT Solution*. 1999; New York:Avery Publishing, 22, 28.

Anderson, G.L.; et al. "Effects of conjugated equine estrogen in postmenopausal women with hysterectomy: the Women's Health Initiative randomized controlled trial." *JAMA*. 2004; 291(14): 1701–12.

Arnot, B. *The Breast Cancer Prevention Diet*. 1998; New York: Little Brown and Company, 35, 96.

Banks, E.; Beral, V.; Reeves, G.; et al. "Fracture incidence in relation to the pattern of use of hormone therapy in postmenopausal women." *JAMA*. 2004; 291(18): 2212–2220.

Barrett-Connor, E. "Hormones and heart disease in women: Where are we in 2005?" *Current Atherosclerosis Reports*. 2006; 8: 85–87.

Barrett-Connor, E.; Grady, D.; Stefanick, M.L. "The rise and fall of menopausal hormone therapy." *Annu Rev Public Health*. 2005; 26: 1–26.

Bland, J. "Cellular communication and signal transduction." *Improving Intracellar Communication in Managing Chronic Illness*. 1999; Gig Harbor, WA: The Function Medicine Institute, 26, 118.

Canonico, M.; Oger, E.; Plu-Bureau, G.; et al. "The estrogen and thromboembolism risk (ESTHER) study. Hormone therapy and venous thromboembolism among postmenopausal women; impact of the route of estrogen administration and progestogens: the ESTHER study." *Circulation*. 2007; 115: 840–845.

Col, N.F.; Pauker, S.G. "The discrepancy between observational studies and randomized trials of menopausal hormone therapy: did expectations shape experience?" *Ann Intern Med*. 2003; 139: 923–929.

Duschek, E.; Neele, S.J.; et al. "Effect of raloxifene on activated protein C (APC) resistance in postmenopausal women and on APC resistance and homocysteine levels in elderly men: two randomized placebo-controlled studies." *Blood Coagulation and Fibrinolysis*. 2004; 15(8): 649–655.

Edmunds, E.; Lundray, M.; Lip, G. "Hormone replacement therapy and intima-media thickness of the common carotid artery: The Rotterdam study." *Stroke*. 2000; 31: 2266–i.

Fugh-Berman, A.; Scialli, A. "Gynecologists and estrogen: An affair of the heart." *Perspectives in Biology and Medicine*. 2006; 49(1): 115–130.

Grady, E., et al. "Cardiovascular disease outcomes during 6.8 years of hormone therapy." *JAMA*. 2002; 288(1): 49–57.

HER Place. "Natural Hormones vs. Synthetic Hormones." http://www.herplace.com/hormone-info/natural-vs-synthetic.htm

Holtorf, K. "The bioidentical hormone debate: are bioidentical hormones (estradiol, estriol, and progesterone) safer or more efficacious than commonly used synthetic versions in hormone replacement therapy." *Postgraduate Med*. 2009; 121(1): 1–13.

Hsia, J.; Margolis, K.L.; Eaton, C.B.; et al. "Prehypertension and cardiovascular disease risk in the Women's Health Initiative." *Circulation*. 2007; 115: 855–860.

Hulley, S.; Grady, D.; Bush, T.; et al. "Randomized trial of estrogen plus progestin for secondary prevention of coronary heart disease in perimenopausal, menopausal, and port menopausal women: Heart and Estrogen/Progestin Replacement Study (HERS) Reasearch group." *JAMA*. 1998: 280; 605–613.

Laux, M. *Natural Woman, Natural Menopause*. 1997; New York: HarperCollins, 8, 20.

Mandavilli, A. "Hormone in the hot seat." *Nature Medicine*. 2006; 12(1): 8–9.

*Mayo Clinic Women's Health Source*. Sept 2002; 3.

Merz, N.B. "Hormone therapy and cardiovascular risk: Why the focus on perimenopausal women?" *Advanced Studies in Medicine*. 2006; (6): 267–274.

Miyagawa, K.; Rosch, J.; et al. "Medroxyprogesterone interfaces with ovarian steroid protection against coronary vasospasm." *Nature Medicine*. 1997; 3(3): 324–327.

Morch, L. "Hormone therapy and ovarian cancer." *JAMA*. 2009; 302(3): 298–-305.

Nelson, H.D.; Humphrey, L.L.; Nygren, P.; Teutsch, S.M.; Allan, J.D. "Postmenopausal hormone replacement therapy: scientific review." *JAMA*. 2002; 288(7): 872–881.

Ridker, P.M.; Hennekens, C.H.; Rifai, N.; et al. "Hormone replacement therapy and increased plasma concentration of C-reactive protein." *Circulation*. 1999; 100: 713–716.

Ridker, P.M.; Buring, J.E.; Shih, J.; et al. "Prospective study of C-reactive protein and the risk of future cardiovascular events among apparently healthy women." *Circulation*. 1998; 98: 731–733.

Rifai, N.; Buring, J.E.; et al. "Is C-Reactive protein specific for vascular disease in women?" *Annals of Internal Medicine*. 2002; 136(7): 529–533.

Rossow, J.E.; et al. "Risks and benefits of estrogen plus progestin in healthy postmenopausal women : principal results from the Women's Health Initiative randomized controlled trial." *JAMA*. 2002; 288(3): 321–33.

Shumaker, S.A.; Legault, C.; Rapp, S.R.; et al. "Estrogen plus progestin and the invidence of dementia and mild cognitive impairment in postmenopausal women." *JAMA*. 2003; 289: 2651–2662.

Stampfer, M.J.; Colditz, G.A.; Willet, W.C.; et al. "Postmenopausal estrogen therapy and cardiovascular disease. Ten-year follow-up from the Nurses' Health Study." *New England Journal of Medicine*. 1991; 325(11): 756–62.

Stark, K.D.; Park, E.J.; Holub, B.J. "Fatty acid composition of serum phospholipids of Premenopausal and postmenopausal women receiving and not receiving hormone replacement therapy." *Menopause*. 2003: 10(5): 448–55.

Van Baal, W.; Kenemans, P.; Van der Mooren, M.J.; et al. "Increased C-reactive protein levels durng short-term hormone replacement therapy in healthy postmenopausal women." *Thrombosis and Haemostatsis*. 1999; 81(6): 925–8.

Wilson, P.W.; Garrison, R.J.; et al. "Postmenopausal estrogen use, cigarette smoking and cardiovascular morbidity in women over 50. The Framingham study." *N Engl J Med*. 1985; 313: 1038–1043.

Women's Health Initiative Steering Committee. "Effects of conjugated equine estrogen in postmenopausal women with hysterectomy." *JAMA*. 2004; 291(14): 1701–1712.

Writing Group for the Women's Health Initiative Investigators. "Risk and benefits of estrogen plus progestin in healthy postmenopausal women." *JAMA*. 2002; 288: 321–333.

Yanick, P. *Prohormone Nutrition*. 1998; Montclair, NJ: Longevity Institute International, 57, 358.

## HORMONAL TESTING METHODS

Bland, J. "Carbohydrate intolerance, insulin, DHEA and oxidative stress." *Nutritional Improvement of Health Outcomes—The Inflammatory Disorders*. 1997; Gig Harbor, WA: The Institute For Functional Medicine, Inc., 81.

Brinker, F. *Herb Contraindications and Drug Interactions*. 2001; Sandy, Oregon: Eclectic Medical Publications, 81–82.

Campbell, B.C.; Ellison, P.T. "Menstrual variation in salivary testosterone among regulatly cycling women." *Horm Res*. 1993; 37: 132–136.

Dabbs, J.M. "Salivary testosterone measurements; reliability across hours, days, and weeks" *Phys Behav*. 1990; 48: 83–86.

Dabbs, J.M.; Campbell, B.C.; Gladne, B.A.; Midgley, A.R.; Navarro, M.A.; Read, G.F.; Susman, E.J.; Sumkels, L.M.; Worturer, C.M. "Reliability of salivary testosterone measurement; a multicenter evaluation." *Clin Chem*. 1995; 41: 1581–1584.

Devenuto, F.; Ligon, D.F.; Friedreichsen, D.H.; Wilson, H.L. "Human erythrocyte membrane. Uptake of progesterone and chemical alterations." *Biochem Biophys Acta*. 1969; 193: 36–47.

Ellison, P., et al. "Measurements of salivary progesterone." *Annals of the New York Academy of Science*. 1993; 694: 161–176.

Finn, M.M.; Gosling, J.P.; Tallon, D.F.; Baynes, S.; Meehan, F.P.; Fotrell, P.F. "The frequency of salivary progesterone sampling and the dx of luteal phase insufficiency." *Gynecol Endocrinol*. 1993; 6: 128–134.

Gozansky, W.S.; Lynn, J.S.; Laudenslager, M.L.; Kohrt, W.M. "Salivary cortisol determined by enzyme immunoassay is preferable to serum total cortisol for assessment of dynamic hypothalamic–pituitary–adrenal axis activity." *Clinical Endocrinology*. 2005; 63: 336–341.

Harris, B.; Lovett, L.; Newcombe, R.G.; Read, G.F.; Walker, R.; Riad-Fahmy, D. "Maternity blues and major endocrine changes: Cardiff puerperal mood and hormone study." *BMJ*. 1994 Apr; 308: 949–953.

Hinchcliffe, C., et al. "Urinary hormones." *Townsend Letter*. Jan 2008; 63–67.

Hirmamatsu, R.; Nisula, B. "Uptake of erythrocyte associated component of blood testosterone and corticosterone to rat brain." *J Steroid Biochem Molec Biol*. 1991; 38: 383–387.

Hofman, T., et al. "Steroid hormones in saliva." *Diagnostic Endocrinol Met*. 1998; 16(9): 265–273.

Koefoed, P.; Brahm, J. "The permeability of the human red cell membrane to steroid sex hormones." *Biochim Biophys Acto*. 1994; 1195: 55–62.

Krzymowski, T.; et.al. "Steroid transfer from the ovarian vein to the ovarian astery in the sow." *J Reprod Fertil*. 1982; 65: 451–456.

Lipson, S.F.; Ellison, P.T. "Development of protocols for the application of salivary steroid analysis to field conditions." *AM J Human Biol*. 1989; 1: 249–255.

Lo, M.S.; Ng, M.L.; Azmy, B.S.; Khalid, B.A. "Clinical application of salivary cortisol measurement." *Sing Med J*. 1992; 33: 170.

Lu, Y.; Bentley, G.R.; Gann, P.H.; Hodges, K.R. "Chatterton RT. Salivary estradiol and progesterone levels in conception and nonconception cycles in women: evaluation of a new assay for salivary estradiol." *Fertil Steril*. 1999; 71: 863–868.

Lu, Y.C.; Chatterton, R.T.; Vogelsong, K.M.; May, L.K. "Direct radioimmunioassay of progesterone in saliva." *J Immunoassay*. 1997; 18: 149–163.

Mandel, I., et al. "The diagnostic use of saliva." *J Oral Pathol Med*. 1990; 19: 119–125.

McCracken, J.; Schramm, W.; Einer-Jenson, W. "The structure of steroids and their diffusion through blood vessel walls in a counter current system." *Steroids*. 1984; 43: 293–303.

Petsos, P.; Reatcliffe, W.A.; Heath, P.F.; Anderson, D.C. "Coparisons of blood spot, salivary and serum progesterone assays in the normal menstrual cycle." *Clin Endocrin*. 1986: 24; 31–38.

Read, G.F.; Walker, R.F.; Wilson, D.W.; Griffith, K. "Steroid analysis in saliva for the assessment of endocrine function." *Ann NY Acad Sci*. 1993; 260–274.

Riad-Fahmy, D.; Read, G.F.; Walker, R.F. "Salivary steroid assay for assessing variation in endocrine activity." *J Steroid Biochem*. 1983; 19:265–272.

Riad-Fahney, L., et al. "Steroids in saliva for assessing endocrine function." *Endocr Rev.* 1982; 3(4): 367–395.

Rosner, W., et al. "Sex hormone-binding globulin mediates steroid hormone signal transduction at the plasma membrane." *Jour Steroid Biochem Mol Biol.* 1999; 69(1–6): 481–485.

Sannika, E.; Terho, P.; Suominen, J.; Santli, R. "Testosterone concentrations in human seminal plasma and saliva and its correlation with non-protein-bound and total testosterone levels in serum." *Int J Andrology.* 1983; 6: 319–330.

Spearoff, L.; Glass, R.; Kase, N. *Clinical Gynecologic Endocrinology and Infertility.* 1999; Baltimore, MD: Lippincott Williams and Wilkins.

Stephenson, K. "The Salivary Hormone Assessment in the Clinical Evaluation of the Female Patient." *International J of Pharmaceutical Compounding.* 2004; 8(6):427–435.

Sumiala, S.; Tuominen, J.; Huhtaniemi, I.; Maenpaa, J. "Salivary progesterone concentration after tubal sterilization." *Obstet Gynecol.* 1996; 88: 792–796.

Swinkels, L.M.; Ross, H.A.; Smals, A.G.; Benraad, T.J. "Concentration of total and free dehydroepiandrosterone in plasma and dehydroepiandrosterone in saliva of normal and hirsuite women under basal conditions and during administration of dexamthathesone and corticotrophin." *Clin Chem.* 1990; 16: 2042–2046.

Vinign, R.; McGinly, R.; Maksvytis, J.; Ho, K. "Salivary cortisol: a better measure of adrenal cortical function than serum cortisol." *Ann Clin Biochem.* 1983; 20: 329–335.

Vining R., et al. "Hormones in saliva: mode of entry and consequent implications for clinical interpretation." *Clinical Chemistry.* 1983; 29(10): 1752–1756.

Vining, R., et al. "The measurements of hormones in saliva: possibility and pitfalls." *J of Steroid Biochem.* 1987; 27: 81–94.

Vliet, E., et al. "New insights on hormones and mood." *Menopause Management.* 1993; June/July: 140–146, 202.

ZRT Laboratories. "Comparative pricing of saliva vs. blood serum hormone testing." Beaverton, OR, 2003.

## SERMs

BreastCancer.org. "SERMs (Selective Estrogen Receptor Modulators)." http://www.breast cancer. org/treatment/hormonal/serms/

Nilsson, S., et al. "Mechanisms of estrogen action." *Physiol Rev.* 2001; 81(4): 1535–1565.

Paruthiyil, S., et al. "Estrogen receptor beta inhibits human breast cancer cell proliferation and tumor formation by causing a G2 cycle arrest." *Cancer Res.* 2004; 6491: 423–428.

## BIRTH CONTROL PILLS

Brownstein, D. *The Miracle of Natural Hormones.* 1998; West Bloomfield, Michigan: Medical Alternatives Press, 11, 54.

Coenen, C., et al. "Changes in androgens during treatment with four low-dose contraceptives." *Contraception.* 1996; 53(3): 171–176.

Murray, M. *The Healing Power of Herbs.* 1995; California: Prima Publications, 375.

Vliet, E., et al. "New insights on hormones and mood." *Menopause Management.* 1993; June/July: 140–146, 242.

Yanick, P. *Prohormone Nutrition.* 1998; Montclair, NJ: Longevity Institute International, 43, 358.

Yarnell, E. *Clinical Botanical Medicine.* 2009; New Rochelle, NY: Mary Ann Liebert, Inc., 13.

## NUTRITION AND HRT

Arnot, B. *The Breast Cancer Prevention Diet.* 1998; New York: Little Brown and Company, 35, 113.

Aten, R., et al. "Ovarian vitamin E accumulation: evidence for a role of lipoproteins." *Endocrinology.* 1994; 135(2): 533–539.

Barnes, M., et al. "The effects of vitamin E deficiency on some enzymes of steroid hormone biosynthesis." *Int J Vitamin Nut Res.* 1975; 45(4): 396–403.

Beattie, J., et al. "The influence of a low boron diet and boron supplementation on bone, major mineral and sex steroid metabolism in post-menopausal women." *Br J Nutrition.* 1993; 49(3): 871–884.

Collins, J. *What's Your Menopause Type*. 2000; Roseville, CA: Prima Health, 181, 192, 204.

Lindeman, R. "Trace minerals: hormonal and metabolic interrelationships." *Principles, Practice of Endocrinolgy and Metabolism*. 1995; Philadelphia: J.B. Lippincott.

Musicki, B. "Endocrine regulation of ascorbic acid transport and secretion in luteal cells." *Bio Reprod*. 1996; 54(2): 399–406.

Naghii, M., et al. "The role of boron in nutrition and metabolism." *Prog Food Nutr Sci*. 1993; 17(4): 331–349.

Omura, T., et al. "Gene regulation of steroidogenesis." *J Steroid Biochem Mol Biol*. 1995; 53(1–6): 19–25.

Reddy, R., et al. "Effects of vanadyl sulphate on ornithine decarboxylase and progesterone levels in the ovary of rat." *Biochem Int*. 1989; 18(2): 467–474.

Shrubsole, M., et al. "Dietary folate intake and breast cancer risk results form the Shanghai Breast Cancer Study." *Cancer Res*. 2001; 61(19): 7136–7141.

Walsh, C., et al. "Zinc: health effects and research priorities for the 1990s." *Envir Health Perspect*. 1994; 102(suppl2): 5–46.

Wolf, C., et al. "Effect of natural oestrogens on tryptophan metabolism: evidence of interference of oestrogens with kyneureninase." *Scand J Clin Lab Invest*. 1980; 40(1): 15–22.

# About the Author

Pamela Wartian Smith, MD, MPH, is a diplomate of the American Academy of Anti-Aging Physicians and director of the Master's Program in Medical Sciences, with a concentration in Metabolic and Nutritional Medicine, at the University of South Florida School of Medicine. An established speaker and author on the subject of wellness and anti-aging, Dr. Smith is also the Director of the Fellowship in Anti-Aging, Regenerative, and Functional Medicine. Currently, she is the owner and director of the Center for Healthy Living, with locations in Ann Arbor, Bloomfield Hills, Grosse Pointe, and Traverse City, all in Michigan, and also in Tampa, Florida.

# Index

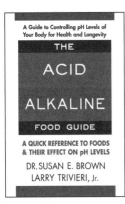

# THE ACID-ALKALINE FOOD GUIDE

## A Quick Reference to Foods & Their Effect on pH Levels

### Dr. Susan E. Brown and Larry Trivieri, Jr.

In the last few years, researchers around the world have reported the importance of acid-alkaline balance to good health. While thousands of people are trying to balance their body's pH level, until now, they have had to rely on guides containing only a small number of foods. *The Acid-Alkaline Food Guide* is a complete resource for people who want to widen their food choices.

The book begins by explaining how the acid-alkaline environment of the body is influenced by foods. It then presents a list of thousands of foods—single foods, combination foods, and even fast foods—and their acid-alkaline effects. *The Acid-Alkaline Food Guide* will quickly become the resource you turn to at home, in restaurants, and whenever you want to select a food that can help you reach your health and dietary goals.

*$7.95 • 208 pages • 4 x 7-inch mass paperback • ISBN 978-0-7570-0280-9*

## TRANSITIONS LIFESTYLE SYSTEM
# GLYCEMIC INDEX FOOD GUIDE

### For Weight Loss, Cardiovascular Health, Diabetic Management, and Maximum Energy

### Dr. Shari Lieberman

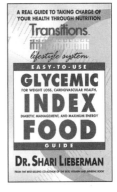

The glycemic index (GI) is an important nutritional tool. By indicating how quickly a given food triggers a rise in blood sugar, the GI enables you to choose foods that can help you manage a variety of conditions and improve your overall health.

Written by leading nutritionist Dr. Shari Lieberman, this book was designed as an easy-to-use guide to the glycemic index. The book first answers commonly asked questions, ensuring that you truly understand the GI and know how to use it. It then provides both the glycemic index and the glycemic load of hundreds of foods and beverages, including raw foods, cooked foods, and many combination and prepared foods. Whether you are interested in controlling your glucose levels to manage your diabetes, lose weight, increase your heart health, or simply enhance your well-being, *Transitions Lifestyle System Glycemic Index Food Guide* is the best place to start.

*$7.95 • 160 pages • 4 x 7-inch mass paperback • ISBN 978-0-7570-0245-8*

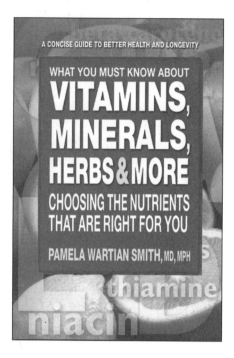

# What You Must Know About Vitamins, Minerals, Herbs & More

Choosing the Nutrients
That Are Right for You

Pamela Wartian Smith, MD, MPH

Almost 75 percent of your health and life expectancy is based on lifestyle, environment, and nutrition. Yet even if you follow a healthful diet, you are probably not getting all the nutrients you need to prevent disease.

In *What You Must Know About Vitamins, Minerals, Herbs & More*, Dr. Pamela Smith explains how you can restore and maintain health through the wise use of nutrients.

Part One of this easy-to-use guide discusses the individual nutrients necessary for good health. Part Two offers personalized nutritional programs for people with a wide variety of health concerns. People without prior medical problems can look to Part Three for their supplementation plans. Whether you want to maintain good health or you are trying to overcome a medical condition, *What You Must Know About Vitamins, Minerals, Herbs & More* can help you make the best choices for the health and well-being of you and your family.

*$15.95 • 448 pages • 6 x 9-inch quality paperback • ISBN 978-0-7570-0233-5*

**For more information about our books, visit our website at www.squareonepublishers.com**